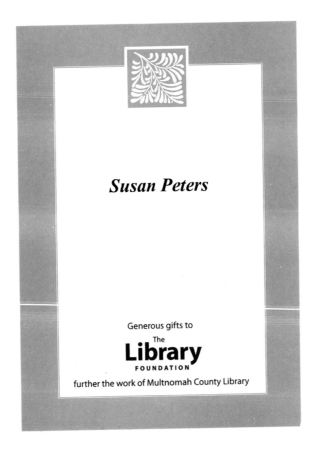

Gold Medal Fitness

ALSO BY DARA TORRES

Age Is Just a Number

GOLD MEDAL FITNESS

A REVOLUTIONARY 5-WEEK PROGRAM

DARA TORRES

with Billie Fitzpatrick

Broadway Books · New York

BROADWAY

Published in the United States by Broadway Books, an imprint of the Crown Publishing Group, a division of Random House, Inc., New York.

www.crownpublishing.com

BROADWAY BOOKS and the Broadway Books colophon are trademarks of Random House, Inc.

Library of Congress Cataloging-in-Publication Data
Torres, Dara, 1967–
Gold medal fitness: a revolutionary 5-week program / by Dara Torres; with Billie Fitzpatrick. —1st ed.
p.   cm.
1. Physical fitness.   2. Weight loss.   3. Conduct of life.
I. Fitzpatrick, Billie.   II. Title.

RA781.T665 2010
613.7—dc22   2010002880

ISBN 978-0-7679-3194-6

Printed in the United States of America

Design by Ralph Fowler/rlfdesign
Photographs by Andrea Mead Cross

10 9 8 7 6 5 4 3 2 1

FIRST EDITION

I wish to dedicate this book to my mom

for all the years of her support, encouragement,

and love, and for the sacrifices she

made to help my dreams become a reality;

and to my daughter, Tessa,

for her continued and neverending

inspiration

Acknowledgments

No book is written alone, and in the creation of this one I have many to thank, including David Hoffman, Michael Lohberg, Anne Tierney, Steve Sierra, Andy O'Brien, Penny Johnson, Chris Jackson, Bruno Darzi, Mark Schubert, Richard Quick, Randy Reese, Terry Palma, and Evan Morgenstein, as well as those throughout my career who have helped me reach my athletic goals.

I would also like to thank Billie Fitzpatrick, my collaborator, who helped me capture in book form what fitness truly means; Christina Malach, my editor at Broadway/Random House, whose focus, energy, and nurturing of this project made all the difference; Diane Salvatore, whose overall publishing vision helped steer this project; Stacy Creamer, for her original belief in this book; Tammy Blake, who has been by my side for both my books, helping them reach all my readers; jacket designer Jean Traina; interior designer Songhee Kim; and Julie Sills for go-to marketing of this book. I'd also like to thank Andrea Cross and Kelly Kwiatkowski of Studio 25 Design for their super photographic artistry.

Contents

Gold Medal Fitness

INTRODUCTION

As an athlete, staying in shape has been my life's work. It's also my passion and the source of my strength and confidence. When I work out, I feel most like myself and most comfortable in my body and mind. I feel motivated to continue to set new goals for myself, go after them, and give them my all. You might think that this tenacity comes from being an Olympic athlete, but I believe it's the result of living in my body in an active way. Working out and staying in shape is simply how I take care of myself, and when I do this, everything else in my life falls into place. The same can happen for you. You might not have come to this book with aspirations to make the Olympics, but I can promise that what you find here will not only show you how to achieve your best physical shape, it will also inspire you to be the best you can be in all areas of your life.

Gold Medal Fitness is a five-week plan that will reshape your body through revolutionary strengthening and resistance stretching exercises that lengthen, tighten, and build your muscles. The plan will also offer a fresh, efficient way to include cardio in your workout, and share what has become my secret weapon—an active recovery phase. This plan is based on the training I've been doing for the past four years, since I made the decision, as a thirty-nine-year-old new mom, to try out for the 2008 Olympic team. Because of these cutting-edge techniques, my own fierce determination, and the support of a handful of devoted trainers, I not only went to Beijing to compete, I came home with three silver medals.

The games in Beijing were my fifth Olympics. My competitive-swimming career has spanned three decades, and I'm not finished yet. As a student at the University of Florida, I earned the maximum possible number of NCAA all-American swimming awards—twenty-eight—and as the first U.S. swimmer to compete in five Olympic Games, I set three world records and won twelve Olympic medals, including four gold. And I'm still not finished.

This book is for all of you who don't want to hang up your suit, take off your running shoes, or give up on feeling—and looking—great. My memoir, *Age Is Just a Number,* might have introduced you to me and some of the events in my life. But this book will share my workout regimen with you. We may not have exactly the same goals, but I bet we do share similar needs. Wouldn't you like to pick up your kids without your back aching? Have the energy for an early-morning workout before getting kids to school or yourself off to work? Achieve a sense of balance that enables you to feel relaxed, confident, and strong instead of depleted by the end of the day? I will show you how to achieve these results—and more—while getting into the best shape of your life.

How This Book Came to Be

After the 2008 Beijing Olympics and the publication of my memoir, I traveled around the country doing a book tour and making appearances as spokesperson for Hewlett-Packard, Fitness Nutrition, and other companies and organizations. During this busy year, as I continued to train for the nationals and World Championships, I met thousands of women and men of all ages who wanted to hear about how I had made a comeback as a forty-one-year-old athlete.

As I crisscrossed the country, I was struck by how many women approached me with questions. "How do you do it?" "I can't believe you're still going so strong! What's your secret?" I began to think about how I approach training and how my regimen might actually help other people—regardless of their age or level of athleticism—get into better shape. Yes, I've been a competitive athlete for a long time, and I probably do have a genetic edge in terms of body type and athletic skill. But I am also just like you—a busy woman and mother, juggling work, child raising, and training (my primary job). And like you, my day doesn't end when I finish training for the day—I also take care of my very active four-year-old daughter. I continue to travel, give talks, and attend book promotions and other sponsor-related events. I'm basically always on the run, trying to keep up with all that I have to do.

The more I thought about how to answer the myriad questions these women (as well as some men) were asking me, the more I realized that across the span of five Olympics, I've never stopped changing, adjusting, and fine-tuning how I train and stay in shape. I think it's this realization that has most inspired me to write this book: I believe that you, too, can achieve optimal fitness if you make getting and staying in shape a priority; adapt your workout routine to your body's ever-changing needs; approach working out as an integral part of taking care of yourself; and then go for it. Training does not mean focusing on one part of your body or group of muscles; it's a full-body experience and approach to taking care of yourself. For all of you women out there who think you might have what it takes to get physically fit—regardless of your age, your shape, your weight, or your long list of responsibilities—you definitely can. But you've got to want it.

In this book I am offering a simple, straightforward plan of exercises and workouts that will strengthen your core and increase your lean muscle mass through dynamic resistance stretching techniques. You will also learn a unique strengthening approach that is absolutely essential for women (especially as women begin to feel the effects of their age) as well as a choice of cardio workouts—all based on the combination that I've been doing with my committed group of trainers. I am now forty-three and probably in the best shape of my life, but these workouts are not just for those of us past forty. In fact, many of my teammates who are in their twenties have adapted these stretching and strengthening techniques and found amazing results—increasing their speed and endurance, recovering from practices and meets more quickly and with less downtime, and bouncing back from injury more fully. These women are elite-level athletes, but like me, they need to constantly work at their overall fitness in order to maintain their strength.

So for those of you who are coming to this book to get in shape, you will find some fabulous tips, exercises, and workouts that will tone you, strengthen you, and make you leaner. You might be twenty-five, thirty-five, or forty-five—but you will see and feel results in just five weeks. Why five weeks? Because it takes most of us that amount of time to learn the proper execution of the strengthening and stretching movements and to see the results.

Some of these exercises incorporate simple pieces of equipment (a Swiss ball, a BOSU Balance trainer, elastic bands, for example), some incorporate gym machines, and others you can do completely on your own.

In many ways this is an anti-program fitness book—because I believe it's crucial to listen to your body and pay attention to what it needs and how it is responding to certain exercises. If your quads feel tight, for instance, you may need to adjust your workout accordingly, stretching both your quads and hamstrings before doing any strengthening. So *you* play a big role in how successful you will be with these workouts. Can I guarantee that you'll have six-pack abs? No, because a big part of making this plan work is up to you. But if you want them, I'll show you how to get them. And if you don't, but instead just want to slim your waist and strengthen your core so that your lower back doesn't bother you, or have more stamina and accuracy when you play tennis, or simply feel better as you get in and out of the car and run through your day (as most women do—kids or no kids), then you'll find that, too. And through some commonsense nutrition advice, you can learn to trim a few pounds if necessary, allowing the hard work you're doing in your training to make more of an impact.

How the Book Works

The book is organized into two parts, with part 1, "You Can Do It!," opening with three chapters. In chapter 1, I will share the story of how I realized I needed to adapt my workout regimen after I turned thirty-five in order to improve my performance and feel better in my body. In chapter 2, I will help you reintroduce yourself to your own inner athlete, a mind-set that will help anchor you and orient you before you begin the workouts. And in chapter 3, "Nourishing Your Body," you will learn more about my approach to eating and taking care of yourself every day. Included in this chapter is a sample meal plan that mimics my weekly diet and tips about how to eat before, during, and after your workout. I will also educate you about the supplements you can add to your daily diet to improve muscle strength, enable your joints to recover, and speed up metabolism. With this information, you will be able to prepare your body—and your mind—for the workouts ahead.

In part 2, "Your Body as Power Source," you will be introduced to

- strengthening exercises in chapter 4, "Strength: The Reason Behind the Ripple";

- resistance stretching techniques (including further strengthening movements) in chapter 5, "Stretching: The Ki-Hara Way";

- options for integrating cardio into your regimen in chapter 6, "Cardio: Why You've Got to Move"; and

- ways to make recovery a conscious part of every workout in chapter 7, "Recovery: The Key to Your Performance."

By the end of these chapters, you will not only understand why these four elements—strengthening, stretching, cardio training, and active recovery—are so essential to any workout, but you will also be familiar and comfortable with the individual exercises that make up the full five-week plan that follows in chapter 8, "Putting It Together."

In the five-week plan, you will find a blueprint of specific routines that includes the basic level of strength movements (progression A), the 17 Ki-Hara resistance stretches, cardio workouts, and active recovery suggestions. It's important that you complete the first five-week block, so that you give yourself time to learn the proper execution of the movements and exercises in order to maximize their impact on your body. Once you have completed the first five-week block, you might feel you need more of a strength challenge and want to progress to the next two five-week blocks that are included, progressions B and C. These blocks include more advanced and challenging strengthening exercises; the stretching, cardio, and recovery tips remain the same.

Throughout the book I will offer boxes of information called "Torres Tips"—advice that I've picked up from trainers and experts throughout my career, little habits I've practiced, and other helpful hints that can make a big difference in your body and mind.

I have tried to make the exercises as straightforward as possible, the suggestions on nutrition and food simple yet delicious, and the overall plan flexible enough to allow you to make working out a regular part of your daily life—all so that you don't have to overthink any part of it. But one thing is for certain: In five weeks you will feel so much better, you will want to continue this plan forever.

Now let's get started.

PART 1

YOU CAN DO IT!

1

GETTING INTO THE FAST LANE, ONE MORE TIME

||||||||||||||||||||||||||||||||||||||||||||||||||||||||||||||||||||||||||||||||||||||||||||||||||||||||||||||||||||||||||||||||||||||

I n the world inhabited by competitive swimmers, I've been considered old for a long time. The first time I really felt this was when I decided to make a comeback for the 2000 Olympic team. I was thirty-two years old, and some people, including my beloved dad, thought I was crazy. He still believed in me, though, as did many other supporters, but the most important factor was that *I* believed in me. I made the team, went to Sydney with my fellow Americans, and won five medals—two gold and three bronze. But who's counting?

That experience was the first time I was forced to relearn how to both push my body and respect it. It was a turning point in my career, and I had to dig deep inside of myself, rethink how to train my body, and ask new questions about what makes a person stronger and more flexible—in body and in mind. In other words, I had to understand how not to let my age get in my way.

I've always had my own sense of time, and in most ways it's worked for me. Most swimmers will tell you that at one point they simply decide to hang up their suit. I've had moments like that, too, but I've reversed my decision now a total of three times. The last such time was when I was thirty-eight and finally, miraculously, got pregnant after years of trying. I jumped back into the pool simply to get some exercise and get rid of morning sickness during my pregnancy, believing that a strong body would only help to make my baby stronger. Being in the pool again felt so right that I was encouraged to begin yet another new training regimen. And two years after my daughter, Tessa, was born, I found myself, at the age of forty-one, in Beijing at my fifth Olympic Games.

As the title of my memoir, *Age Is Just a Number,* indicates, I like to challenge the odds. I believe that most of us can not only reach beyond our own preconceived limitations but also rise to challenges much bigger than we allow ourselves to dream . . . *if* we simply believe in ourselves. I know that's a big if. How do you gain that trust in yourself? By setting up real, measurable goals and developing realistic expectations and plans to meet those goals. Then, of course, there's follow-through. Don't expect to lose those last five or ten pounds if you're not consistent with your workouts. Don't expect to run that 5k if you haven't been running 3 miles three or four times a week. Don't expect to finish that book you've always wanted to write if you don't sit down at the computer several times a week. Results demand showing up. However, it's also true that when you do show up and put in the work, you might just exceed your own expectations.

So, when I put on my Speedo and my old goggles again, I knew that as a thirty-nine-year-old new mom I had to train differently. I couldn't expect that my body was the same as it was in Sydney six years earlier, or in Barcelona eight years before that. Once I understood this, I learned three very important lessons: (1) I needed to develop more flexibility so that my muscles and joints were more balanced and supported one another; (2) I had to strengthen my body in a new way (lean and long rather than bulky and beefy); and (3) most important of all, I had to recognize the importance of recovery for my mind and body. These three elements combined to make me a faster, stronger, and smarter swimmer. Rest and recovery time, functional strength training, and resistance stretching have been my mantra, my secret weapons, and the key not only to competing as a forty-something athlete but also to feeling amazingly confident and comfortable in my body. And they can be yours as well—just wait and see.

Lesson Number One: Know When to Back Off

Although on the surface motherhood didn't seem to change my body, it did make an enormous impression on me, especially in one unforgettable way: It taught me how to pay attention to what my body needed. It was becoming clear to me that I couldn't push my body until it ached with pain; I couldn't *not* eat well before and after workouts; I couldn't sleep off a too long training session—because now I had a daughter, Tessa, to take care of.

These differences became even more apparent after I was back in the pool and had begun to seriously prepare and train for the Beijing Olympics in 2008—almost two years away. I could tell that my body was reacting differently than it had before. I was used to pushing myself to the max, and now I felt tired after a long workout. I was used to a certain level of physical discomfort, but now my doctors were telling me to take better care of my joints, especially my knees and shoulders. I was not recovering as easily or quickly. I felt weighed down by bulky muscles. I knew I should do things differently, but I had no idea how or what to do. Then I remembered part of what I learned back at Stanford.

When I was training for the 2000 Sydney Olympics with my then coach Richard Quick, I had learned the hard way not only that comparing myself with other swimmers, especially much younger swimmers, gets in the way of training and swimming my best but that becoming unnecessarily focused on what you can't control (i.e., another swimmer's performance or training style) can drag you down. At the time, I had an active and rather charged rivalry with swimmer Jenny Thompson. We'd been teammates and friends, but when I moved to Stanford to train with Richard Quick and the rest of the team, hoping to make the Olympic training camp and trials, I got caught up in a competition that was incredibly stressful.

I also found myself comparing my workout with what the twenty-year-olds were doing in the pool and at the gym. At the time I thought, "If I don't do what they're doing, how am I going to make the team? If I don't swim as long, I'll never get better results." For me, not winning is never an option. But I was confused as to what to do, how to adapt.

It was Richard who told me to back off. "You need to rest, do you understand that?" he said to me one day after practice. It was Friday and I was pooped.

I kind of nodded, hoping he would just stop talking to me.

"Really, you need to rest. For real. I don't want you doing one thing this weekend. Not even one."

Through his glare, I knew he was serious and meant every word. What he was saying was true.

So that weekend, against every grain in my body, I rested. I resisted the urge to do a spin class, run—or swim. And by the end of the weekend, I actually felt better than I had in months. That Monday I swam one of the best practices of my life. I had learned my lesson: I needed to let my body recover when it needed to.

This experience made me realize that I didn't necessarily have to train more than the other athletes but I had to train smarter. That's what being the oldest woman on the team meant: I had to conserve my energy, use it more wisely, so I could exert it more powerfully. Again, the most important element of this was about recovery. How do you actively recover? You let your body rest, you disengage your mind from its constant thinking, and you RELAX. This has a huge and positive impact on your performance when it's done right. Active recovery also means eating a balance of whole foods from all the food groups (carbs, protein, and fat, with plenty of fiber), but not getting too hung up about how much you eat. Recovery also means replacing fluids, electrolytes, and amino acids that fortify you—mind and body.

As an older athlete, I know that when I don't allow myself to recover, I don't swim as fast, move as fluidly, or feel as good—in and out of the pool. But when I do work in that essential time to recharge my body, I feel totally in sync with myself. My mind and body are attuned to each other, and I trust myself more. Trust is a big factor—the older we get, the less we can use the "push through the pain" mentality. Instead we need to replace it with learning to listen to our body's signals. When you've allowed your body to recover, you can trust it—you know when to push it, when to rest it.

Lesson Number Two:
Become Strong and Smart

The next lesson I learned about training as an older athlete was how important it is to develop strength—but in a way that at the time was completely new to me. I learned this lesson from an amazing strength coach named Andy O'Brien. When I met Andy, I didn't quite understand his approach to strength building. He wasn't at all impressed that I could bench-press 205 pounds. In fact, he let me know right away that all my muscle-bound bulk was probably slowing me down in the pool. He also pointed out that the swimmer ripping up the pool with the biggest guns is often not the one who reaches the wall first.

I was introduced to Andy serendipitously through the general manager of the Lexus dealership near my house in Florida. As Tessa and I were waiting for my car, the manager came up to me and said he'd read a recent Mother's Day article about my decision to try to make the 2008 Olympic team. And as if he was reading my mind, he told me about another client of his who happened to be the strength trainer for the Florida Panthers hockey team. Hockey? What did that have to do with swimming? But I took Andy's number and figured it couldn't hurt to give him a call.

On the phone, I told Andy about my swimming career and what I could do in a weight room, and in his charming and easygoing Canadian way, he let me know he had something else in mind. It was immediately clear to me that Andy was going to offer me something more, something very special indeed.

When we met for lunch the next day, Andy explained in a simple, concise way that muscle speed, which I needed for swimming, comes from highly coordinated movements and fluid timing. Weight training, which developed as a form of static bodybuilding, is not meant or designed to create much movement. Think of those old-fashioned poses of bodybuilders flexing their muscles for the camera or a line of judges. You can't quite imagine them springing into action.

Andy's approach was all about teaching the body to become strong and balanced so it can move as efficiently as possible. This meant instead of bulking up, I needed to become leaner, enabling my muscles to move quickly. He said the type of exercises he could teach me would train my muscles to react quickly and to move in coordination with other muscle groups. A main focus was around the core, which included not only the abdominal muscles but also the lower back and the chest. Andy explained that a strong, supple core—one

Stretch to Strengthen

Gym rats love to bulk up their muscles and call themselves strong. But can they move? If you can't move your body with ease, if you can't touch your toes and move from side to side easily and lightly, then strength doesn't matter. You've got to *strengthen* and *stretch*!

that could move with the rest of my body—was essential to increasing my range of motion. When you work out muscles through three planes of motion (I'll explain more about this concept in chapter 4), you maximize your body's fitness.

Needless to say, as soon as I understood how Andy's approach worked, I signed on to train with him. First he watched me work out in the gym, taking careful inventory of my strengths and weaknesses, looking at how I was using my strong muscles to compensate for my weak ones. Next he analyzed how I swam—how my strokes impacted my upper body, how my lower body reacted to that movement, and how much speed I generated from my legs as well as my arms. Once he was through observing me and getting to know my body, he came up with a specific training regimen, which he said he would then change every five weeks so my body wouldn't plateau.

Andy also talked about how he had to rehabilitate me (he actually used that word!) by doing all sorts of crazy drills. His first goal was to straighten and balance me out, and he had to do this discretely, letting my muscles learn new patterns of movement without a lot of weight attached at the other end.

I felt the results of Andy's training approach in less than a week. My body felt more buoyant in the water, and I was able to move more fluidly and quickly. After about four weeks, I began to see my body change:

The bulk was lessening, and my muscles became leaner and longer. And when I swam in my first competitive event, it was clear: I was faster.

Lesson Number Three: Get Flexible

The third lesson I learned about being an older athlete is that I needed to stretch. Before the 2000 Olympic trials, I had never integrated any kind of real stretching routine into my training. For me, as with most swimmers, stretching entailed doing a pinwheel with my arms, and maybe attempting to touch my toes and circle my wrists. But my coach at the time, Richard Quick, suggested I do Pilates. One day while I was working out on the Pilates Reformer machine, I noticed two guys in white shirts doing some kind of strange bodywork on a woman who looked like an athlete. Intrigued, I watched them manipulate the woman's legs and arms, getting her limbs and joints to move at what looked like might be painful angles. I was curious.

"What are they doing over there?"

"That's what you really need," my Pilates instructor said.

"What do you mean?" I asked, thinking, "No way am I going to do that."

"I promise you—it's what you need. When we're done here, you should go talk to those guys."

But I knew she was probably right. Besides, the Pilates didn't seem to be working enough to strengthen my core and stretch my body.

So after my Pilates session I approached the two trainers to find out more about what they were doing. I learned that their technique was called resistance stretching, and it was totally different from any stretching regimen I'd ever seen.

To be honest, I wasn't exactly eager to try it. It looked too weird. But I knew that as an older athlete I needed to stay open to new ways of sustaining my body. I asked for the stretchers' phone numbers and thought I'd give them a call the next day. What could it hurt?

That was more than ten years ago, and I've been doing resistance stretching ever since. I began working with a man named Bob Cooley, but after I finished competing in Sydney, I started working with two amazing trainers, Steve Sierra and Anne Tierney, who are still with me today. The more I understood their approach and felt the results, the more convinced I was that stretching, especially resistance stretching, needed to be an essential part of my training routine. Stretching made a huge difference in how my body moved on land and in the water. Steve and Anne practice a form of resistance stretching called Ki-Hara—a blend of stretching and strengthening that not only maximized my swim workouts but made an enormous impact on my overall physique.

Ki-Hara is about creating balance and efficiency in the body. By moving and stretching the body in ways that mimic how a body moves in real life, which means in multi-joint and multi-movement rotations, you can increase your flexibility and your range of motion. In ways similar to what I was doing with Andy's strength exercises, which incorporate three planes of movement, Ki-Hara works the muscles with the joints in ways that add strength, flexibility, balance, and co-ordination. It is crucial, especially as we age, that body movements are both smooth and safe. When we move—whether during athletics or everyday life—it's not always possible to protect our joints. Ki-Hara teaches the body how to contract the muscles while being lengthened in ways that are most effective and at the same time prevent injury. Essentially, Ki-Hara trains the muscles the way they are used most frequently: eccentrically.

Think of stretching your hamstrings or quads like you would a rubber band. In order to get the most power and speed (the two necessary components and objectives of swimming and many other sports such as running) from your major muscles such as your hamstrings, you need to strengthen them *as* you stretch them. The muscles need to be able to contract and extend with the same efficiency and ability. Later I will go into more detail about how stretching is also a matter of contraction (or concentric motion) and relaxation (eccentric motion). For now, what you need to know is how different this approach to stretching sounded to my ears at the time.

Steve and Anne's exercises work for elite athletes and weekend warriors as well as those of you who are just beginning a workout routine after time (even years!) away. Ki-Hara can help any body function better as a whole by teaching you how to move safely and without pain. It is low-impact and great for people of all ages, abilities, and fitness levels because you tailor the resistance to fit your needs.

With Andy's strength training, Ki-Hara resistance stretching, and the active recovery I was now so conscious of, my body became stronger and more fit and my reaction time in the water improved. In a very short period, I was swimming better and faster, and recovering more quickly and completely. I felt so much healthier—I not only lost about ten unnecessary pounds (that bulk that Andy had commented on!) but also felt leaner and smarter about how I was working my body.

This kind of improvement in my overall fitness level had more than just physical effects. I also felt my confidence grow. Of course, I was never without nerves and anxiety before a competitive event or swim meet, but something inside of me felt more centered, more secure. Because my body was so balanced, I could trust it more, which enabled me to relax more before competitions. I might have achieved this equilibrium anyway, given my years in the sport, but I believe that these three changes in my training approach at this juncture of my life were really at the heart of this peace of mind and renewed belief in myself.

I feel the positive impact of this in every aspect of my life: I'm a more patient, grounded mother and a more self-assured woman and professional. Again, I've learned the lesson that when I take care of my body, when I strengthen it from the inside out, I make myself stronger as a person. And I believe that the same will happen for you.

I sure wish I'd known some of what I know now when I was in my twenties. It's never too late, of course, but if you are now in your twenties or thirties and think that some of the recovery business just doesn't apply to you or that stretching is for dancers and yoginis, think again. Some of my twenty-year-old teammates have become conscious of these elements of training—and wow, have they benefited! The strengtheners that Andy has taught me—and that I have shared here—are so powerful, you will see results in your body in just four to five weeks. Your skin will become tighter, your muscles will become leaner and more toned, and your silhouette will become slimmer because you will have lost inches. You will feel remarkably more energetic and good in your clothes. And as you incorporate the resistance stretching exercises, you will reinforce the leanness of your muscles as they become more pliable and flexible. When these targeted techniques strengthen the muscles around your joints, enabling more fluid movements, walking through your day will feel so much easier.

This is what fitness really boils down to: feeling good inside your skin and in your clothes, trusting that you can get out of bed with a spring in your step, and enjoying an active, fun-filled life.

2

YOUR INNER
ATHLETE

I was born competitive. I don't just want to win in the pool—I want to win in life. What does this mean? It means that when I was younger, everything—from piling into the car for school to calling my mother first on her birthday—was a competition with my siblings. I love the challenge and promise of a win. I love the excitement and rush of pushing myself to the edge. But more than anything, I love a good race. That was true when I was eight years old, and it's still true now at forty-three.

As I was first thinking about writing this book, I realized that many of you might not share this insane need to win or compete, but where I think we are all quite similar is in the fact that we feel much better about ourselves—inside and out—when we push ourselves toward a goal. Being an athlete, many of my goals involve my body—pushing it, training it, imagining it accomplishing a number of mini-goals before reaching the ultimate goal (the 50-meter freestyle, making the national team to qualify for Worlds, the Olympics—whatever the specific goal is at the time). For me, naming my goals, being clear about them, and, most important, knowing what steps I need to take in order to accomplish the goals has played a huge role in the successes I've enjoyed. I'm a planner, and I have learned a crucial lesson: When you plan out each detail of how to accomplish a goal—create a road map, so to speak—you absolutely better your chances for reaching that goal. And if you don't plan, you will often be met with failure.

I've been lucky enough to live out the childhood dreams of many girls and young women, and I can't stress enough the positive impact this has had on all aspects of my life. So many women stop playing sports after high school or college—some even earlier. Studies show the positive correlation for girls between sports and high self-esteem, between sports and good grades and later success, and between sports and the avoidance of drugs, alcohol, and other kinds of trouble. So it gives me pause to think of all that is lost when girls become women and stop running around playing sports and enjoying their physicality.

This is one of the major benefits of getting in and staying in shape: The more active you are physically, the more you will feel connected to your body. You will take better care of yourself, your health will improve, and your self-esteem will increase. So even if you have lost that playground spark, it's not too late to get back out there and make physical activity fun for you.

I want to challenge you to rediscover that part of yourself. The part that loved running a race on the blacktop of your school yard, that joined the softball team and loved cheering for your friends as they rounded the bases (even if you sometimes closed your eyes in the outfield when a high ball came your way). It might take a while to shrug off the cobwebs and relearn how to be spontaneous and natural in your body. It might at first be uncomfortable to let yourself feel a desire to win a race. But one of the purposes of this five-week fitness plan is to give you the permission and the opportunity to do just that: be that little girl again who wants to win and achieve a goal—just for the heck of it.

Establishing Your Goals

So I'd like to ask you: What are your goals in reading this book? Obviously, you don't have to compare your goals with mine, and you also don't have to compare your goals with your sister's, your best friend's, or your neighbor's. Goals are uniquely personal commitments to yourself. Perhaps you want to train for a breast cancer walk or lose five pounds and keep them off.

Read the following questions before determining your goals. In fact, I suggest you get some kind of journal or notebook, a place where you can jot down some thoughts (you can use it later to keep a record of your workouts).

For now, read through the questions and give yourself some time to consider your answers. If you rush into naming specific goals, the tendency is to be unrealistic. Of course you don't want to set the bar too low, but it's easy at the outset of a new fitness program to want to get to some results too quickly.

Say you want to lose some weight and go down a dress size or two for a friend's wedding that's coming up. If the wedding is two months away, is it realistic to expect yourself to lose twenty pounds? Wouldn't you be happy to lose ten and go from a size 14 to a size 10 or 12? Or perhaps you've always wanted to run a marathon but haven't been running for a number of years; you might want to set up some goals that are more realistic—maybe start with a 3k or 5k race.

It's important to be realistic about your expectations so you don't set yourself up to fail. Keep in mind that once you get to chapter 8, "Putting It Together," you will be asked to review your goals before starting your five-week plan. At that point, you may have a clearer sense of what your goals are and match them with what will make your dreams a reality.

Identify Your Fitness Goals

Deciding upon goals takes focus and clarity. These questions will help you determine where you are now and where you want to be—in terms of your current health, your habits, and your desired fitness. Read through these questions; then go through them one by one and respond to them in a journal or an online notebook.

1. What about yourself would you most like to change?

2. When was the last time you had a complete physical and learned your cholesterol, BMI (body mass index), and protein levels?

3. How often are you sick in a year?

4. Focus in on your current physical condition:

    a. **Cardiovascular:** Are you able to walk up a flight of stairs with ease?

    b. **Muscle strength and endurance:** Can you do a push-up? If so, how many at one time?

    c. **Balance and coordination:** Can you stand on one foot without losing your balance?

d. **Flexibility:** Are you able to touch your toes? Are you able to turn your head fully to the right and left? Do you have any pain or lack of motion in your joints?

5. How much time are you willing to devote to your fitness program?

6. Write down your specific health and fitness goals:

   a. **Health goals:** For example, do you want to lose or gain weight? Do you want to reduce your cholesterol? Increase your lean muscle mass and decrease your fat?

   b. **Fitness goals:** For example, do you want to learn to play a new sport, enter a walkathon, or compete in a race or tri-athlon? Do you want to be able to finish a spin class?

   c. **Mind/body balance goals:** How are you dealing with stress in your life? How many hours of sleep do you get each night? Do you ever have trouble falling asleep or waking in the middle of the night, unable to fall back to sleep?

   d. **Downtime:** Do you get enough time to enjoy your family? Your partner? Yourself? How often do you see friends socially?

7. Have you ever tried to accomplish similar fitness goals in the past? Were you able to follow through?

   a. If you answered no, explain what got in your way. You might want to think about how and why a program you did in the past didn't work for you. Was it your lack of commitment? Boredom? Too little time?

8. Are you determined to eat a more nutritious diet? What, if anything, might you change about the way you eat?

9. Do you know what is required of you to accomplish the goals you are now setting for yourself? Do you need some more advice? A specific eating and workout plan? How much do you rely on external structure to stick to a plan?

10. Take a moment and think about when you can incorporate four to five 45- to 60-minute workouts each week. You don't have to commit yet. But keep your schedule in mind, so that when it's time to get started, you have a basic plan.

By identifying your goals and keeping them clear in your mind, you strengthen your chances of accomplishing them. But remember to listen to your body. Once you begin working out, your body will tell you how it feels, but it's up to you to pay attention and respect the message. If you're feeling sluggish and can't focus at work, then you might be working out too strenuously. If you feel slightly sore but otherwise good, you are probably working out just enough. Let your goals inspire you, but know that they may need to be adjusted according to how your body responds.

Tapping into Your Confidence

Like anyone, I wake up some mornings not wanting to practice—not even wanting to get out of bed. I get tired and weighed down by the long list of things I have to do every day. And sometimes I feel self-doubt. I am not a robot. I'm sure you have days like these, too. The trick to keeping your mind focused and your drive fresh is to get into the habit of tapping into your reservoir of confidence—a deep and

Find a Doctor You Like

Finding a doctor you trust and see regularly (at least once a year) to make sure that you're in good health is one of the key elements of fitness. I consult doctors as soon as I feel that something isn't right. In the past, I would wait and wait, just hoping I could work through the pain—but often I would end up with an injury. I've finally learned that I'm more apt to seek medical advice if I actually like the person dispensing it. If you don't like your doctor, how can you expect yourself to go regularly? It's crucial that you find a physician or nurse practitioner with whom you feel comfortable so you're more likely to ask all your questions and check in on an annual basis. Here's a quick list of tests you should ask for annually .

1. Cholesterol

2. Blood sugar

3. Protein

4. Vitamin D

5. Blood pressure

6. BMI

7. Iron

8. Allergies or food sensitivities, including to gluten and dairy*

* You may not need to test annually for potential food sensitivities, but many people are reactive without realizing it.

nurturing well that you will learn to replenish each time you reflect on your accomplishments.

You will naturally feel more confident the more you work out. Doing the strength and stretching exercises, as well as integrating cardio into your workout routine, will not only make you physically strong but mentally stronger, too. If you find yourself losing steam or coming up with excuses not to work out, then you need to pause and focus on the negative thought cycle that may be developing.

If you pay attention, you might catch yourself thinking negative thoughts:

"I'm too tired. I need to sleep."

"I'll never make it anyway. Why even try?"

"I'm just not a born athlete."

These negative thoughts can take on more power if you don't stop them in their tracks. If you simply become aware of their negative, self-defeating nature, then you give yourself the opportunity to make a choice: Do you really believe that you're too tired to work out? Do you really believe that you have to be a "born athlete" in order to benefit from becoming more fit? Do you really believe that it's only the end result that matters? Giving these false beliefs a second thought will no doubt lead you to see how they are mere distractions, not obstacles to you reaching your goals.

Mental Strength

Over the years I've developed a kind of armchair philosophy for keeping myself mentally strong based on some commonsense advice I've learned from coaches, trainers, other athletes, and my own experience. This isn't hard science, but it works for me, and I think it might help you as well:

1. **Keep your focus.** It's fine to let your mind wander when you're shopping or cleaning your house, but when you work out or practice your sport, try to keep your mind attuned to what you are doing. The more presence of mind you bring to each exercise, the more your mind can enhance your body, especially in the initial part of the movement.

2. **Stick to your routine.** The more you follow your schedule, the more your body and mind get accustomed to the routine, which in turn helps you reinforce and strengthen your commitment—to your goals and to yourself.

3. **Practice.** Every athlete knows that without practice, you can't expect to play well on game day. Practice breeds trust. Practice breeds muscle memory. Practice hones your skills. Practice enables you to battle your nerves on game day.

4. **Do your best.** This tip is about doing your best not just during a performance or competition but during practice. Give each practice, each workout, your all. Don't back off on yourself. Don't tell yourself that you'll run longer, play more intensely, or swim harder the next day. Give it your all every time, and when it's game day or competition day, the intensity of your practice will pay off.

5. **Manage the pressure.** Our nerves can get the best of us. When you feel yourself getting too anxious about your performance, take a deep breath and look off into the distance to shift your attention away from the nervous feeling. Really look at that tree on the right, that bird in the sky, or the gorgeous guy on the treadmill. Let your mind shift so you can take your body away from your anxiety. The feeling will pass if you let it.

6. **Develop a strategy.** The more comfortable and familiar with the individual exercises you become, the more you will be able to direct your workout. For instance, if you are a runner, you might want to do more quad stretches and strengtheners. If you're a swimmer, you might want to practice fast-twitch movements.

Create Your Winning Team

Do you have a colleague who goes to the same gym you go to? Do you have a good friend who likes to do the elliptical before or after work? Is there another mom in your neighborhood who wants to train for an upcoming charity walk or run? Working out with a partner can boost your spirits and increase your results by adding a touch of competition.

I know two women triathletes who have trained together and been best friends for years. Their common love of sports and their camaraderie helps them stick with their training and stay on track, always excited about what they're doing. Two other women I know met when they signed up for a 60-mile, three-day walk for breast cancer. They spent two months doing long walks around their town, forming a bond that kept them motivated and helped them get ready for the day of the event without fear.

I love my support team, feel their encouragement, trust in them without a doubt, and know they trust me. I enjoy winning races and medals for them as much as for myself. This team approach to accomplishing your goals might work for you, too. Once you've established your goals, share them with one or two people you trust and who want you to succeed—maybe your partner, your best friend, your child, a colleague. All it takes is a team of one to bolster your spirits and cheer you on.

7. **Be efficient with your energy.** Don't lollygag through your workout. Most of what I suggest in the pages ahead can be done quickly: The resistance stretches take about twenty minutes; most of Andy's strengtheners can be done in thirty minutes; and the cardio workouts range in time from thirty to forty-five minutes. If you only have an hour for a workout, then you need to manage your time; this will not only make sure you fit in the workout but also make you use your energy (physical and mental) more wisely.

8. **If you feel tired, ill, or injured, back off.** Pushing through pain or working out even though you're coming down with a cold will backfire. Let your body rest when it needs rest. When you take care of yourself by refueling and getting more sleep, you will end up feeling more connected to your body.

9. **Create your own support team.** Another way that I keep my spirits up and my eye on the prize, so to speak, is by surrounding myself with a posse of people who believe in me, who cheer me on, who trust me and help me stay focused. This group includes my mom, my siblings, and, on a daily basis, my trainers. I couldn't be where I am without them. You might not need a team of trainers like me, but everyone can use some support. Reach out to those you trust and tell them of your new fitness plan. Share your goals with them so they can cheer you on. Who knows, you might inspire one of them to join you!

10. **Relax and have fun.** It's easy to get caught up in winning. I've been there, done that—for years. But practice and working out can be something you enjoy and look forward to—not just something you look forward to finishing. And if you let yourself relax while you work out, you might just have more fun!

3

NOURISHING YOUR BODY

||||||||||||||||||||||||||||||||||||||||||||||||||||||||||||||||||||||||||||||||||||||||||||||||||||||||||||||||||||||

When I travel to give speeches or presentations, many of the questions that women ask me have to do with my eating disorder, which I battled over a five-year period in my mid to late twenties. It was one of the biggest challenges I've ever faced. Back at the University of Florida, swimming for the college team, I picked up some bad habits. I was what the experts call a mix of an exercise anorexic (someone who works out to burn calories eaten) and bulimic. Many girls and women in my audiences have shared that they identify with me for various reasons. Some had full-blown eating disorders, including bulimia or anorexia; others have told me about being obsessed with food intake and counting calories; and others have said they spent years binging and purging. We now know that millions of women suffer from some sort of disordered eating, and I feel strongly that we need to help one another stop getting so hung up on food, our weight, and the American obsession with being skinny.

Eating disorders are not only physically debilitating, they are also mentally and emotionally draining and dangerous. It took me a number of years to develop the courage to seek and find help, mostly through therapy, but with that help I was finally able to break the self-sabotaging cycle, and now my disordered eating is a thing of the past.

Recovering from this truly deadly disease changed my life, not only because I stopped purging, which is so unhealthy for your body, but because through therapy, I relearned how to have a natural, easygoing relationship with my body and with food. So if you've come to this book for diet advice, you might be disappointed. I am not a dieter. I don't even like the word. What I am is interested in health and eating foods that taste good, that are good for me, and that give my body and mind essential nutrients to perform at their best.

In this chapter you'll find some general advice on what to eat on the days of your workouts and in your everyday life. I don't draw a big distinction between my workout eating style and non-training style. If I'm training harder as a big competition approaches, I may eat more but just more of the same foods I'm already eating.

In general, I am not a fussy eater, and like many of you I don't have the time or patience to plan my meals ahead of time. I choose simple snacks and meals that are easy and quick to prepare (what a surprise!) but are high on taste. And since most of us don't enjoy preparing more than one meal at a time, these meal plans are also designed to appeal to most kids and are hearty enough to satisfy your partner as well.

When I go out to eat or bring home takeout, I try to keep my food as clean as possible, staying away from processed foods and eating plenty of fruit, vegetables, nuts, and beans. After I've fed Tessa, given her a bath, and gotten her into her PJs, I'm pooped. So when dinner rolls around, I don't have the energy to do anything elaborate. Sometimes I order in Japanese food that's not too salty or fried (I don't "do" fish, so sushi is out for me); I might make a lasagna and make the leftovers last as long as possible. If I have a friend over, I'll consult my (very small) box of recipes and whip something up, always keeping food simple and clean, without a lot of sauces, butter, or salt—all sources of hidden calories and food triggers.

In the pages ahead you'll find a thirty-five-day (five-week) eating plan to accompany the five-week workout plan that comes later in the book. This meal plan is simple and requires virtually no recipes. Each day includes a healthy balance of your main food groups, so you'll be getting enough protein, complex carbohydrates (including fiber!), and essential fatty acids to support both your workouts— and the development of lean muscle mass—and weight loss, if that is your goal.

You will also find a guide to which supplements to take. Regardless of your age, everyone should supplement their vitamin and mineral intake because we cannot get everything we need from food. I get most of my supplemental vitamins through an amino acid drink I have after workouts—a fast, easily digested way to make sure I'm covered. But for those of you who prefer to take capsules, you'll find here all the guidance you need and then some.

The better you eat, the better you will feel—both in your body and in your mind. So consider the information that follows an important step in taking care of yourself, and one that sets the foundation for the workouts that will get you to Gold Medal fitness.

Your Attitude Toward Food and Eating

Like I said, it's easy to get obsessed with food in our culture—we are surrounded by fast food that is filled with empty calories and inundated with media photos and suggestions that send us the message

Good Versus Bad Fats

Not all fat is bad. In fact, our brains and bodies need certain fats in order to function properly, and since our bodies don't produce these essential fatty acids, we need to get them from other sources, such as fish oil, flaxseed, and olive oil, for example. However, we also need to avoid the so-called bad fats that clog arteries, add weight, and put our bodies at risk of disease.

Good (unsaturated) fats: olive and canola oils, peanut butter, macadamia nuts, fish, and avocados

Bad fats: any saturated (butter, cream) or trans fats and partially hydrogenated oils

that we have to be thin in order to be considered attractive. And recently we're being given more information about the hazards to our health of eating nonorganic, processed foods. It's a wonder we all don't throw up our hands and park ourselves on the sofa with a pint of Ben & Jerry's!

So one of the first pieces of advice I want to share with you is this: Relax. Easier said than done? Not really. The more you exercise and commit to being active in a daily way, the more mind-body balance you achieve, and the more relaxed you will feel. What this boils down to: One of the best ways to get control of your food and your thoughts about food is by exercising. You will feel better in your skin; your cravings for sugary foods will naturally decrease; and as you feel more connected to your body, you will naturally gravitate toward foods that are cleaner. What do I mean by clean foods? Foods like fruits, vegetables, and whole grains that are rich in fiber.

They clean the toxins out of your body, speed up your metabolism, and burn away fat.

Here's my healthy-eating mind-set in a nutshell:

- Eat small meals and/or snacks regularly so you don't get too hungry.

- Exercise regularly so your body craves healthy, clean foods and rejects sugary, starchy, processed foods that slow you down.

- Remember to treat yourself so you don't trigger a craving or a binge!

Make Food Easy: Some Basic Guidelines

Easy Guide to Food Groups

I'm not a dietitian, but after all these years being around trainers, nutritionists, and physicians, I've picked up some basic nutritional information that is sound, scientifically supported, and, best of all, easy to live with. In order for our brains and bodies to function, we need to eat foods from the three main food groups—carbohydrates, protein, and fat. Eating these in the right balance is key to good health. I've marked those food categories that you should include and those that you should limit in your diet:

- Protein that is low in fat—lean meat, poultry, seafood, and tofu/soy — **Include**

- Complex carbohydrates that are high in fiber—whole grains, vegetables, and fruit — **Include**

- Legumes—such as beans and lentils—which are a mix of complex carbs and protein and are rich in fiber. These pack a nutrient-rich punch without the fat of meat — **Include**

- Simple carbohydrates—these carbohydrates contain high starch and/or sugar and are low in fiber—found in white breads, pastas, white rice, potatoes, and sweets — **Limit**

- Dairy—milk, cheese, and yogurt are a good source of protein but also tend to be high in fat; always choose non- or low-fat — **Limit**

- Good fats—fats that contain no trans fat and are low in saturated fat and high in omega-3 fatty acids—olive oil, canola oil, fish oil, nuts, and seeds — **Include**

In general, I make sure all meals contain a balance of protein, fat, and carbohydrates (again, these carbs need to be high in fiber). Soluble fiber is a substance natural to fruits, vegetables, beans, and whole grains that not only slows down the absorption rate of food but also fills you up—I like to think of fiber as the magical food that allows us to eat as many fruits and vegetables as we like. It also cleanses the body of toxins, keeps our metabolism working properly, and moves the food in and out with ease. As most nutritionists will tell you, getting fiber in your diet is one of the simplest ways to ensure that your body stays clean and light.

As you become familiar with these food categories, you will find it easier to make healthy food choices. Things get less straightforward and murkier, however, when you turn to processed or packaged foods.

The biggest reason behind the national obesity and diabetes crisis is our overconsumption of processed foods. These products are no longer strictly made up of foods from the three food groups but have added ingredients that literally don't occur in nature. In order to increase the shelf life and add flavor to packaged foods, processed foods are prepared with additives; trans fats, sodium, and other harmful chemicals are included, adding empty calories and stressing our immune systems. The bottom line? Our bodies have no use for and are not meant to metabolize the ingredients added to foods that keep them "fresh" on the grocery-store shelf, in the freezer, or in the cupboard. Try to eat fresh foods as much as you possibly can. And if you have to eat at a fast-food chain or from a package, make your choices wisely. Some fast food is relatively clean and healthy—instead of fried, go for grilled; skip the fries; and try to include a salad for fiber. Even though packaged foods can be overly processed, including all sorts of sodium and chemical additives, there are brands that are organic and/or healthy. The key is to look at the label of any packaged or frozen food and make sure that the sodium count is between 0 and 500 milligrams per serving, that no MSG (monosodium glutamate) is included, and that there are as few artificial colors, sweeteners, or chemicals listed as possible.

Portion Sizes

My guidelines for portion sizes are basic and once you get familiar and comfortable with them, and you stick to eating healthy foods, then you don't really have to worry about calories—you will automatically stay within the range for weight loss and/or maintenance, if that is a concern for you. Most people find it easier to think of their foods in portion sizes, but the only foods that you really need to limit are protein and fats and those carbohydrates that are not high in fiber. There is no limit to how much fruit and vegetables you can eat! But you decide how you want to handle this decision. Some people like the guidelines; others prefer to restrict just the protein and fat and starchy carbs, eating as much of the vegetables and fruits as they like.

As you can imagine, I am not the type to measure, weigh, or over-think my food. Instead, I eyeball amounts and then simply see how I feel. If I'm still hungry, I'll eat more; if I feel full, I'll stop eating. I let my body tell me what it needs. The following guidelines are based on healthy portion sizes that provide enough food to keep you satisfied. If you wish to lose a couple of pounds, these amounts will help you trim calories and reinforce the impact of your workouts so that you lose weight safely.

Here are some basic rules of thumb to follow each day:

- **Protein—fish, chicken, meat, and legumes:** You should limit your protein intake to one piece of meat or fish about the size of your palm and twice that for legumes.

- **Complex carbohydrates—fruits, vegetables, and whole grains:** The portion size for whole grains should be two hand-fuls; but you can eat veggies and fruit to your heart's content. They are so loaded with fiber and vitamins, and act as a natural detox on your body, that you can't eat too much—your body will utilize every ounce. You may also want to try other whole grains such as quinoa, barley, and whole-wheat pasta. I've also suggested Ezekiel toast for breakfast; this whole-grain bread is high in fiber and is a good source of protein.

- **Simple carbohydrates—white bread, pasta, potatoes, cous-cous, and white rice:** Keep your portions of these starchy grains to one fist if it's an accompaniment or two fists if it's the main dish (for example, rice topped with stir-fried veggies).

- **Unsaturated fats:** Limit yourself to one to two tablespoons of peanut or other nut butter or olive or canola oil (for example, in a salad dressing).

Beware of Caffeine!

Did you know that for performance athletes, caffeine is considered a "controlled or restricted" substance by the International Olympic Committee? Caffeine is a stimulant that alters your body chemistry. Despite this warning, many athletes are hooked on high-caffeine drinks such as Red Bull. Thankfully, I've never developed a need for caffeine and in general stay away. You might just want to try what it feels like to go caffeine-free.

- **Dairy:** Milk, yogurt, and cheese are excellent sources of protein and calcium, but you do have to watch the amount of fat they contain. Try to stick to 1-cup portions of low- or nonfat yogurt and ½-cup portions of low-fat milk or cheese. Eggs are also a great source of protein and iron—try to buy organic!

Beverages

Whether your goal is to improve your fitness, lose pounds or inches, or both, it's important to keep well hydrated. However, you need to be conscious and choosy about what you drink. I don't drink coffee or alcohol (I just never developed a taste for either), but I know I am not in the majority. If you drink soda (I do enjoy a frozen Coke every once in a while), iced tea, or green tea, just watch the chemical intake, the sugar, and the flavor substitutes. I drink diet soda, but I try to limit myself to one or two a week. Despite the ongoing research into the best and safest artificial sweetener, the jury is out and I'd rather be safe than sorry. Water is always best!

Eat Breakfast

You've been hearing this since you started kindergarten, right? It's still true: Don't skip breakfast. Kids think better, perform at a higher level, and maintain healthier weight when they eat breakfast, and so do adults, especially adults who have high expectations of themselves.

I love starting my morning meal with a fruit smoothie, so you will see a number of breakfast smoothie suggestions in the meal plan. In general, I use 1 to 2 cups of ice, a mix of fruit that measures about 1 cup (but can really be as much as you want), and some low-fat yogurt or soy milk for a milky texture. I suggest adding a shot of wheatgrass or soy protein powder to add some extra nutrients. Since I swim

TORRES TIP

Miscellaneous Meal Tips

- Any time I recommend dairy (milk, cheese, yogurt, mayonnaise, or ice cream), go with low-fat.
- Any time I include rice, it can be either brown or white rice, but know that brown rice has more fiber.
- Any time I include bread, try to go for whole grain or wheat over white, again because the darker the bread, the more fiber it contains.
- Condiments such as ketchup, mustard, and mayonnaise should be limited to 1 tablespoon—they tend to be loaded with fat and/or sugar.
- Don't add salt to foods if you don't have to.

first thing after waking up five days a week, this breakfast shake literally fuels my muscles and joints.

Take a look at the breakfast suggestions later in the chapter. There should be enough variety to inspire even the most reluctant among you—and your body will thank you for the pre-workout boost.

Supplements

The most important supplement I take on a daily basis is Fitness Nutrition Amino Acid Complex, a rich blend of many amino acids that provides essential building blocks for the body that most of us don't get from our diet. My coach, Michael Lohberg, was the one who got me hooked on amino acids. He said that older athletes need to not only replace the proteins their bodies utilize but supplement them for strength and speed. The combination of vitamins, minerals, and amino acids has increased my energy and endurance, helps me burn fat and build lean muscle mass, improved my performance, and aided my recovery time. This product (which I happily endorse) is amazing. Give it a try! (See www.4fitnessnutrition.com.)

Sufficient vitamins and minerals help boost metabolism, strengthen your immune system, and protect you from many age-related conditions (such as heart disease, diabetes, and osteoporosis). I recommend that everyone, regardless of your age, take four main supplements that will support your workout, make you healthier all around, and assist in weight loss, if that's your goal.

These supplements are:

- **Multivitamin**

- **Omega-3 (EPA and DHA) fatty acids**—found in fish oil or ground flaxseed oil

- **Probiotic**—a beneficial bacterium that protects the body from disease; a great way to keep your GI tract in balance, as well as fight off everyday illnesses

- **Calcium, magnesium, and vitamin D**—most of these are contained in a multi, but not in a sufficient dosage for women over thirty to maintain bone health, improve metabolism, and fight against the effects of aging

Eat Often!

I tend not to eat three square meals a day, opting for several small meals instead. I need a quick pick-me-up snack after a workout (maybe a yogurt, smoothie, or some nuts), and then usually about an hour later I'll eat lunch. I don't eat any heavy meals, but always try to have some protein and pair it with some kind of vegetable, salad, or fruit. If I really want a burger, for example, I'll skip the bun to have some fries, and add a green salad. Or I'll have a Caesar salad with grilled chicken. I watch what I eat, but I eat often.

The point is, you never want to go four hours without eating; you will start to "bonk" (i.e., hit low blood sugar and either feel tired and cranky or trigger a craving for "comfort foods" that usually are fatty and starchy or both). In the meal plan that follows, you will find a lot of suggestions for good snacks.

Dessert

I have a sweet tooth, but I consider anything with refined sugar (chocolate, candy, ice cream) a treat, so I'm always mindful of when I do eat something sweet, which is usually every night after dinner. I am of the

Snack Tips

As I've mentioned, if you don't want to trigger overeating or cravings for sugary or starchy foods, it's best to eat every four hours. Since I eat dinner on the early side, around five or six P.M., having one snack per day usually works for me. But those of you who prefer to eat later in the evening might need to eat a second snack between lunch and dinner.

Here's a quick list of healthy snacks you should have on hand:

- Raw almonds, cashews, or other nuts
- Fresh fruit—apples, pears, peaches, grapes, watermelon, cantaloupe, oranges, bananas
- Raw veggies—carrots, celery, peppers, cucumbers
- Low-fat cheeses in small portions, such as Laughing Cow or mini Bonbel
- Small containers of low-fat yogurt or cottage cheese
- Dried fruit, including apricots, cranberries, and raisins
- Granola

school that if you restrict too much, you might overindulge later. At the same time, I know that if I eat too much sugar in any given day, I feel it. I become sluggish. So allow yourself some sweet treats if that's what you desire, just keep them in moderation.

I did not include a dessert menu in the meal plan; I leave that up to your discretion. But be wise. Don't throw away all your physical work by having a pint of ice cream. Here's a quick list of my favorite desserts or sweet treats.

- Fruit: anytime, anywhere, any kind—it's all good!

- High-quality chocolate

- Ice cream bars—Klondike has one on a stick that's only 100 calories, and I always love an ice cream drumstick!

- Popsicles, Fudgsicles, Skinny Cow, and homemade Rice Krispies Treats (made with spray-on Pam instead of butter)

Salads and Dressings

As you read through the meal plan, you will note that I've included a green salad with many lunches and dinners. You can't eat too much salad! For me a green salad is a bunch of red or green leaf lettuce, chopped romaine lettuce, or Bibb lettuce when it's in season and available. I don't always include tomatoes, carrots, or cucumbers but I know these are popular items, so definitely include them if you wish. In terms of dressing, a good rule of thumb is to limit oil, whether it's olive, canola, or part of a premade dressing, to 1 tablespoon. There are now available many great varieties of store-bought dressings that are actually healthy—with no MSG and little sugar. Stock up on a variety, so that your salad never tastes boring!

When out at restaurants, use your best judgment. Always ask for the dressing on the side or you can expect your lettuce drowned. You only need a bit for flavor, so experiment with bottled dressings or make your own with a dash of a good olive oil and balsamic vinegar.

35 Days of Meals

Day 1

Breakfast
Pancakes (for added fiber, sprinkle batter with
1 tablespoon wheat germ) topped with 1 tablespoon syrup
or jam

Snack
Fruit smoothie with 1 to 2 cups fruit, 1 cup yogurt, ice, and a
shot of wheatgrass or soy protein powder

Lunch
Green salad with grilled chicken and 1 tablespoon your choice
of dressing

Dinner
Stir-fried vegetable medley, including onions, red or green
peppers, zucchini or yellow squash, over brown rice or quinoa
with a side of steamed broccoli

Day 2

Breakfast
Cheese omelet (use 1 egg or 3 egg whites and ½ ounce low-
fat cheese) with 1 tablespoon salsa

Snack

Handful of almonds and a banana or an apple

Lunch

Burger (beef, turkey, or veggie), no bun, with fruit salad. (And watch the ketchup or mayo, using only 1 tablespoon of either if you desire.)

Dinner

Pasta primavera: pasta of your choice with fresh seasonal vegetable combinations, such as squash, peppers, onions, eggplant, and broccoli, with canned tomatoes. In any primavera combination, you can stir-fry the veggies using a spray-on oil or 1 tablespoon oil, or simply steam them.

Day 3

Breakfast

1 cup low-fat yogurt with ⅓ cup granola and 1 tablespoon honey

Snack

Banana

Lunch

Greek salad: romaine lettuce, Kalamata olives, tomatoes, red onion, and ½ ounce feta cheese; topped with 1 tablespoon each olive oil and red wine vinegar, or 1 tablespoon bottled dressing of your choice

Dinner

Grilled salmon, chicken, or shrimp with rice pilaf and asparagus (grilled or steamed)

Why Add Wheatgrass?

Wheatgrass cleanses the body, increases energy and stamina, boosts the immune system, and is high in calcium, magnesium, potassium, phosphorus, and iron!

Day 4

Breakfast

Peanut butter and jelly on whole-wheat or multigrain bread

Snack

Popcorn with Smart Balance butter spray and no added salt

Lunch

Pita bread stuffed with hummus, raw or roasted peppers, and tomatoes and a green salad with dressing of your choice

Dinner

Chinese takeout: stir-fried veggies and chicken over rice

Day 5

Breakfast

Oatmeal with 1 tablespoon honey or maple syrup

Snack

Apple

Lunch

Caesar salad with 1 tablespoon dressing with grilled chicken

Dinner

Chicken noodle soup (canned is fine, but select a brand that is low sodium) with a whole-wheat or multigrain roll and green salad

Day 6

Breakfast

Omelet (use 1 egg or 3 egg whites) with ½ ounce low-fat mozzarella cheese and tomatoes

Snack

½ cup red grapes

Lunch

Turkey sandwich on whole-wheat or multigrain bread with lettuce, tomato, and low-fat mayonnaise

Dinner

2 lentil tacos (lentils, shredded Monterey Jack cheese, salsa, and 1 tablespoon avocado) in soft flour or corn taco shells

Day 7

Breakfast

2 slices Ezekiel bread with 1 tablespoon Smart Balance and/or all-fruit spread

Snack

Fruit smoothie with 1 to 2 cups fruit, 1 cup yogurt, ice, and a shot of wheatgrass or soy protein powder

Lunch

Chef salad: 1 slice each of ham, turkey, and Swiss cheese, 1/2 avocado, 1 hard-boiled egg, a handful of turkey-bacon chips, and 1 tablespoon dressing of your choice

Dinner

Grilled chicken or fish, steamed broccoli, and half a baked potato or whole sweet potato

Day 8

Breakfast

Whole-grain cereal with 1/2 cup low-fat milk and 1/3 cup berries

Snack

Apple slices with peanut butter (1 tablespoon)

Lunch

Tomato soup with a whole-wheat or multigrain roll

Dinner

Turkey meat loaf and green salad with 1 tablespoon dressing of your choice

Day 9

Breakfast

1 cup low-fat yogurt with 1/3 cup granola and 1 tablespoon honey

Snack

Handful of almonds

Lunch

Tunafish salad (made with 1 tablespoon low-fat mayo, chopped red onion, chopped celery, and chopped pickle) on a bed of greens or whole-wheat or multigrain toast

Dinner

Thai takeout: pad Thai

Day 10

Breakfast

Whole-grain cereal with ½ cup sliced bananas and ½ cup low-fat milk

Snack

Grapefruit or orange

Lunch

Grilled salmon over rice with grilled vegetables

Dinner

Filet of beef with side of steamed spinach and half a baked potato

Day 11

Breakfast

Pancakes (for added fiber, sprinkle batter with 1 tablespoon wheat germ) topped with 1 tablespoon syrup or jam

Snack

Handful of almonds or cashews

Lunch

Turkey sandwich on rye bread with lettuce, tomato, and
1 tablespoon mayo

Dinner

2 lentil tacos (lentils, shredded Monterey Jack cheese,
salsa, and 1 tablespoon avocado) in soft flour or corn taco
shells

Day 12

Breakfast

Oatmeal with ¼ cup raisins

Snack

Fruit smoothie with 1 to 2 cups fruit, 1 cup yogurt, ice, and a
shot of wheatgrass or soy protein powder

Lunch

Tunafish salad (made with 1 tablespoon low-fat mayo,
chopped red onion, chopped celery, and chopped
pickle) on a bed of greens or whole-wheat or multigrain
toast

Dinner

Roasted chicken thighs with garlic over rice (rub
fresh garlic on the chicken and place in an ovenproof
casserole in a preheated 425°F oven for 45 minutes until
crispy)

Day 13

Breakfast
2 slices Ezekiel bread with 1 tablespoon Smart Balance and/or all-fruit spread

Snack
2 pieces Laughing Cow low-fat cheese and handful of low-salt Wheat Thin crackers or Triscuits

Lunch
Caesar salad with 1 tablespoon dressing with grilled chicken

Dinner
Breakfast for dinner—breakfast quesadillas: 2 scrambled eggs, 1 tablespoon Monterey Jack cheese, scallions, 1 tablespoon salsa, half an avocado in a whole-wheat tortilla

Day 14

Breakfast
Whole-grain cereal with ½ cup fruit of your choice and ½ cup low-fat milk

Snack
1 cup low-fat yogurt with ⅓ cup granola and 1 tablespoon honey

Lunch
Green salad with nuts, dried cranberries, and orange slices, with 1 tablespoon dressing of your choice

Dinner
Chicken fajitas with rice and/or beans

Day 15

Breakfast
Whole-grain cereal with ½ cup low-fat milk and ⅓ cup berries

Snack
Popcorn with Smart Balance butter spray and no added salt

Lunch
Burger (beef, turkey, or veggie), no bun (top with 1 tablespoon ketchup, mayo, or mustard, if desired), and fruit salad

Dinner
Pasta with pesto sauce, and a green salad with dressing of your choice

Day 16

Breakfast
2 slices Ezekiel bread with 1 tablespoon Smart Balance and/or all-fruit spread

Snack
Pineapple chunks and cottage cheese (or yogurt)

Lunch
Pasta fagioli (pasta with bean soup)

Dinner
Grilled chicken with lemon and orzo with asparagus (grilled or steamed)

Day 17

Breakfast
Pancakes (for added fiber, sprinkle batter with 1 tablespoon wheat germ) topped with 1 tablespoon syrup or jam

Snack
Fruit smoothie with 1 to 2 cups fruit, 1 cup yogurt, ice, and a shot of wheatgrass or soy protein powder

Lunch
Green salad with grilled chicken, with 1 tablespoon dressing of your choice

Snack
Handful of walnuts

Dinner
Stir-fried vegetable medley (broccoli and carrots, zucchini and yellow squash, red, yellow and orange peppers) over rice or quinoa

Day 18

Breakfast
Cheese omelet (use 1 egg or 3 egg whites and ½ ounce low-fat cheese) with 1 tablespoon salsa

Snack
Handful of almonds and a banana or an apple

Lunch
Spinach salad with ½ ounce goat cheese, a handful of walnuts, and mandarin orange slices

Dinner

Burger (beef, turkey, or veggie), no bun (top with 1 tablespoon ketchup, mayo, or mustard, if desired), and fruit salad

Day 19

Breakfast

1 cup low-fat yogurt with ⅓ cup granola and 1 tablespoon honey

Snack

Banana

Lunch

Greek salad: romaine lettuce, Kalamata olives, tomatoes, red onion, and ½ ounce feta cheese; topped with 1 tablespoon each olive oil and red wine vinegar

Dinner

Grilled salmon, chicken, or shrimp with rice pilaf and asparagus (grilled or steamed)

Day 20

Breakfast

French toast made with multigrain bread, dipped into 1 egg or egg white, topped with 1 tablespoon Smart Balance spread or syrup

Snack

1 cup low-fat yogurt

Lunch

Pita bread stuffed with hummus, raw or roasted peppers, and tomatoes and a green salad with dressing of your choice

Dinner

Chinese takeout: stir-fried veggies and chicken over rice

Day 21

Breakfast

Oatmeal with 1 tablespoon honey

Snack

Apple

Lunch

Chicken noodle soup, whole-grain roll, cucumber and tomato salad, 1 tablespoon each olive oil and red wine vinegar

Dinner

Pasta arrabiata: penne with crushed tomatoes and red pepper flakes (the key is to prepare the pasta al dente, then add the tomatoes and pepper flakes; cook for 2 minutes) and a green salad with 1 tablespoon dressing of your choice

Day 22

Breakfast

Omelet (use 1 egg or 3 egg whites) with ½ ounce low-fat mozzarella cheese and tomatoes

Snack

½ cup red grapes or 2 slices watermelon

Lunch

Turkey sandwich on whole-wheat or multigrain bread with lettuce, tomato, and 1 tablespoon low-fat mayonnaise

Dinner

Poached halibut topped with chopped cherry tomatoes and basil, served with steamed green beans and side of rice. (To poach fish, place in a Pyrex baking dish with ½ cup water, cover tightly, and bake in a preheated 425°F oven for 20 minutes or until fish is cooked through.)

Day 23

Breakfast

2 slices Ezekiel bread with 1 tablespoon Smart Balance and/or all-fruit spread

Snack

Fruit smoothie with with 1 to 2 cups fruit, 1 cup yogurt, ice, and a shot of wheatgrass or soy protein powder

Lunch

Chef salad: 1 slice each of ham, turkey, and Swiss cheese, ½ avocado, 1 hard-boiled egg, a handful of turkey-bacon chips, and 1 tablespoon dressing of your choice

Dinner

Grilled chicken breast with steamed broccoli and half a baked potato or whole sweet potato

Day 24

Breakfast
Whole-grain cereal with ½ cup low-fat milk and ⅓ cup berries

Snack
Apple slices with peanut butter (1 tablespoon)

Lunch
Tomato soup with a whole-wheat or multigrain roll

Dinner
Roast turkey with steamed green beans and half a baked potato

Day 25

Breakfast
1 cup low-fat yogurt with ⅓ cup granola and 1 tablespoon honey

Snack
Handful of almonds or cashews

Lunch
Tunafish salad (made with 1 tablespoon low-fat mayo, chopped red onion, chopped celery, and chopped pickle) on a bed of greens or whole-wheat or multigrain toast

Dinner
Thai takeout: pad Thai

Day 26

Breakfast
Oatmeal with ¼ cup raisins

Snack
1 slice Ezekiel bread with 1 tablespoon Smart Balance and/or all-fruit spread

Lunch
Bean and barley soup (canned is fine, but select a brand that is low sodium)

Dinner
Gnocchi (potato dumplings) with marinara sauce, a green salad with 1 tablespoon dressing of your choice, and side of asparagus (grilled or steamed)

Day 27

Breakfast
Bowl of multigrain cereal with ½ cup sliced bananas and ½ cup low-fat milk

Snack
Grapefruit or orange

Lunch
Grilled salmon over rice with grilled vegetables

Dinner
Italian restaurant: appetizer-sized pasta with green salad (dressing on the side) and sautéed spinach

Day 28

Breakfast
French toast made with multigrain bread, dipped into 1 egg or egg white, topped with 1 tablespoon Smart Balance spread or syrup

Snack
Banana or apple

Lunch
Japanese restaurant: edamame, miso soup, California roll

Dinner
Pasta with pesto with pine nuts and a green salad with 1 tablespoon dressing of your choice

Day 29

Breakfast
2 scrambled eggs (or 3 egg whites) with 1 tablespoon salsa

Snack
Apple

Lunch
Turkey club (low-sodium turkey, 2 strips turkey bacon, lettuce, tomato, 1 slice low-fat cheese, 2 slices whole-wheat bread with a little mustard or nonfat mayo)

Dinner
Rice and beans; green salad with fresh tomatoes and cucumbers

Day 30

Breakfast
2 slices Ezekiel bread with 1 tablespoon Smart Balance
and/or all-fruit spread

Snack
Popcorn with Smart Balance butter spray and no added salt

Lunch
Chicken fajitas

Dinner
2 lentil tacos (lentils, shredded Monterey Jack cheese, salsa,
and 1 tablespoon avocado) in soft flour or corn taco shells

Day 31

Breakfast
Fruit smoothie with 1 to 2 cups fruit, 1 cup yogurt, ice, and a
shot of wheatgrass or soy protein powder

Snack
Low-fat cheese or hummus on multigrain crackers

Lunch
Green salad with grilled chicken slices, tomatoes, and
1 tablespoon dressing of your choice

Dinner
Beef tacos (use 90 percent lean beef, crispy corn taco shells,
1 tablespoon salsa, and 1 tablespoon low-fat yogurt instead of
sour cream, and top with shredded lettuce)

Veggies Galore

The key to not getting bored eating vegetables is to try new ones and vary the ones you do eat. Here's a list of easy-to-prepare and highly nutritious vegetables. Remember, these are loaded with fiber, vitamins, and minerals! They naturally hydrate you and fight against the effects of aging.

- Broccoli or broccolini—great sautéed with garlic and olive or canola oil
- Cauliflower—chopped up with garlic and cooked under the broiler—delicious!
- Green beans—I like them steamed al dente
- Edamame (soybeans)—steamed with a bit of salt
- Zucchini and yellow squash—great grilled or sautéed quickly
- Cucumbers—great raw
- Celery—great raw
- Spinach—sautée with garlic, or toss baby spinach in a salad or on a sandwich. When I sautée spinach, I use Smart Balance spray for a bit more flavor.
- Yellow, red, and orange peppers—these are sweet and delicious raw
- Carrots—nothing's better than a raw baby carrot!

I try to eat as many raw vegetables as possible. As soon as a vegetable is cooked, it loses some of its nutritional value. Since having Tessa, I find it easier to eat raw veggies—I cut them up for her and eat some myself.

Day 32

Breakfast
Whole-grain muffin with 1 teaspoon Smart Balance and a slice of cantaloupe

Snack
½ cup red grapes or 2 slices watermelon

Lunch
Turkey burger on a whole-wheat bun with 1 slice of low-fat cheese, lettuce, tomato, and 1 tablespoon mustard, low-fat mayo, or ketchup

Dinner
Grilled salmon topped with 1 tablespoon low-fat yogurt mixed with dill, steamed asparagus, and a green salad with 1 tablespoon each olive oil and red wine vinegar

Day 33

Breakfast
Cheese omelet (use 1 egg or 3 egg whites and ½ ounce low-fat cheese)

Snack
Handful of cherries

Lunch
Burger (beef, turkey, or veggie), no bun, with a green salad and 1 tablespoon dressing of your choice

Dinner

Pasta fagioli (pasta with bean soup) with a whole-wheat or multigrain roll

Day 34

Breakfast

Oatmeal with 1 tablespoon honey or maple syrup

Snack

Banana

Lunch

Green salad with tomatoes, carrots, 2 tablespoons chickpeas, and 1 tablespoon dressing of your choice

Dinner

Grilled shrimp with sautéed broccoli and side of brown rice made with chicken stock instead of water for extra flavor

Day 35

Breakfast

2 slices Ezekiel bread with 1 tablespoon Smart Balance and/or all-fruit spread

Snack

2 pieces Laughing Cow low-fat cheese and handful of whole-grain crackers

Lunch

Chicken quesadilla made with low-fat cheese, salsa, ½ avocado, and ½ cup black beans

Dinner

Filet of beef with side of steamed spinach and half a baked potato

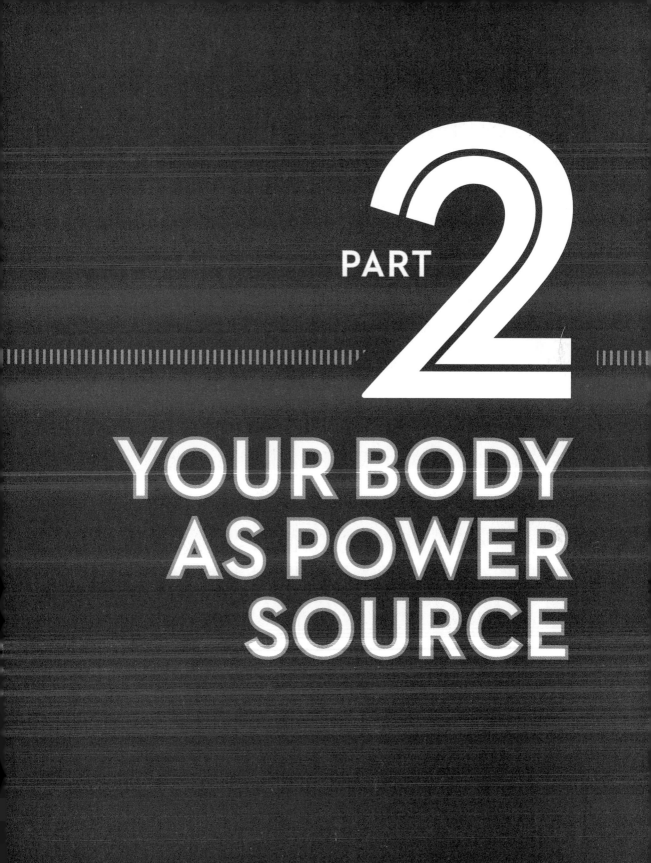

PART **2**

YOUR BODY AS POWER SOURCE

4

STRENGTH
The Reason Behind the Ripple

|||||||||||||||||||||||||||||||||||||||||||||||||||||||||||||||||||||||||||||||||||||||||||||||||||||||||

When I met Andy O'Brien, I could bench-press 205 pounds. He wasn't impressed. In fact, he implied that I was a meathead, or at least that I looked like one. He didn't exactly use those words, but that seemed to be the point.

The day I met Andy, we had agreed to have lunch at my favorite diner near my house. Always early, I was sitting at a table with my coach, Michael Lohberg, when a young, fresh-faced guy approached.

"Hey, Dara, I'm Andy."

Without hesitating, I shot back, "Are you even twenty yet?" But I was soon going to learn that Andy's youthful appearance belied the depth of his knowledge.

As soon as I heard Andy describe his approach to strength training, and understood his philosophy, I was hooked. Long, lean muscles. Efficiency and speed. Joint protection. Increased stability. Core strength multiplied by ten. He had me at hello.

What Andy Taught Me

My coach has always told me that one of my assets as an older athlete has been my stability. What is stability? It's your body's ability to stay grounded and aligned during movement, which is by and large a function of strength. Andy shared a great story with me about the Olympic gymnast Olga Korbut. For those of you who remember this petite powerhouse (and for those of you who don't, I'm sure you can catch a video of her in motion on YouTube), you might recall her incredible acrobatic manipulations of her arms, legs, trunk, and spine. At the ripe age of twelve or thirteen she seemed as if she was as flexible as a contortionist in the circus.

Apparently, however, she wasn't flexible as much as she was hypermobile (i.e., she had a greater-than-normal range of motion). And as soon as she stopped training at an elite level and lost muscle mass, her joints went berserk. For many years, she was hobbled by arthritis and could barely move, much less bend. Swimmers are often hypermobile and consider their youthful ability to rotate their arms in their shoulder sockets proof of everlasting flexibility. Unfortunately, this is often a false flexibility. The key to harnessing the mobility is strengthening the muscles around the joints and making them stable.

This was one of the primary ways that Andy helped me. When I began working with him, he seemed to be exposing weaknesses I didn't even know I had, which really got under my skin. I could barely do even the simplest exercises with minimal weight. For example, using five-pound dumbbells and carving letters in the air—a *T, W, V, M,* and *J*—with each arm while balancing on a Swiss ball felt arduous. But as I learned to focus on my core and use it to cue into my balance, I began to feel different in my body. And it showed in the water. After only four weeks, I broke a U.S. Masters record.

In a way, Andy retaught me how to think about my body: from my head to my toes, from my bones to my muscles and even my joints. He showed me how, as a swimmer for more than thirty years, I had overdeveloped my front chest muscles and how my middle back was actually weak. With any imbalance, a strong part of your body will compensate for a weaker one. After doing a careful inventory of the ways I used my body and then watching me swim, he came up with a series of movements that literally changed the way I moved, strengthened muscles I barely knew I had, stabilized the muscles around my joints, and basically put my body back into balance. The exercises helped me focus on my core, realign my skeleton, and strengthen the muscles around my joints, making me more stable. They also helped stimulate my nervous system so that my muscles worked more fluidly in coordination. One specific result that I noticed right away was that my fast-twitch muscle reflexes were much faster.

And although I have always had big shoulders and narrow hips, my abs didn't always look the way they do now. I will say without a doubt that Andy's workout is the supreme reason behind the ripple.

The long-term results? I swam faster, I looked leaner, and I felt better than I had in years. I've worked with Andy for more than three years now. He has helped me hone those original exercises, and I still do the simplest ones religiously. For this book, Andy has helped me outline five groups of movements that work on the three planes of

TORRES TIP

Think Like a Dancer

Andy taught me to think of each exercise as if it were a dance movement, paying exquisite attention to its execution and doing it with grace, not robotically. This way, I slow down, focus, and maximize the benefits of each movement. It's important to always go slowly in the first part of an exercise; you need to take your time in order to get it right and give it your full intensity.

movement. And they all stem from and strengthen the core. The more comfortable you become with the exercises, the better you will move from a singular plane of movement to multiple planes.

The Anti-Plan

It was because of Andy that I decided that I didn't want this book to offer a plan that reduced what I did to a program that anyone could follow without thinking. What differentiates Andy's approach to strength training from other methods is that it asks you to pay attention to the subtleties of each movement and how your body is responding. If you line up five people and ask them all to do a squat using only their own body weight as resistance, you will probably see five different versions. One person might be leaning too far back in her heels; another might lean too far forward with his weight in his feet; a third might have her knees outside of the line of her toes; and a fourth might have overdeveloped quads and weak hamstrings and so use the stronger muscles without ever strengthening the weaker ones, or vice versa.

If you do an exercise without giving thought to proper alignment and without awareness of your own deficiencies or imbalances, then you will never right the wrong. If, however, you focus on each of the movements and learn to do them correctly, then over a short period of four to five weeks you will not only strengthen your weaknesses, you will also bring your interrelated muscle groups (and joints and bones) more into balance. What's important at this point—before beginning the workouts themselves—is that you start believing in their ability to really change your body. These exercises can and they will—but you've got to make it happen.

Andy has helped me design five groups of three exercises (for a total of fifteen movements) that will enable you to strengthen your core (including your back, chest, and abs), your legs, and your arms—all while maximizing your efficiency, alignment, and stability.

First, you will learn discrete movements that strengthen your core, using only one plane of movement; gradually you will incorporate more complex movements that combine two planes of movement (biplanar), and finally you will progress to a workout that includes strength training on three planes of movement (multiplanar).

At the same time, you'll be varying the speed or tempo of certain exercises to create more of a challenge and sometimes an aerobic component. Another way to ramp up the challenge, especially for your balance, is to integrate an unstable surface for some of the exercises. Of course, this requires that you be completely aware of and comfortable with the proper execution of each movement.

You will be using some equipment such as a Swiss ball, a BOSU trainer, and a medicine ball as well as gym machines, including an elliptical, treadmill, and various weight machines. You will learn how to engage your core in each movement, whether it's a plyo push-up, a body squat, or an incline press.

Together, these exercises will help build your body's strength while training it to move efficiently, conserving energy and protecting it from injury. The movements build on one another, so that as you become more proficient and move from singular-plane movements to biplanar movements to multiplanar movements you progress from simple to more complex. And as you do the movements, you are engaging more and more muscle groups and joints and using more motions—mimicking how you move in everyday life and in sports.

All of the movements are described with simple instructions and accompanied by photos of me doing them. At first, the exercises may seem deceptively simple. As I said earlier, when I first started doing them I felt kind of awkward, unsure of how these micro movements were going to make me stronger. My coach, Michael Lohberg, actually thought they were downright silly. But they worked and they worked well. They have become the mainstay of my strengthening regimen, and the beautiful thing is that they can be performed by people at any level of fitness.

Before starting the exercises, it's beneficial to get acquainted with some key elements that underlie this form of strength training:

- You will start most movements from an athletic stance.

- Isolate your core so you can position your body in alignment and understand how far-reaching your core really is (i.e., it includes not only your abdominal muscles, both high and low, deep and superficial, but also your back, pelvis, groin, and chest).

- Understand that each of the individual movements involves three components:

  - **Efficiency**—each exercise requires careful execution in accordance with biomechanical principles

  - **Progression**—each group of exercises progresses in terms of complexity, increasing the degree of rotation, speed, or level of resistance

  - **Dynamics**—each exercise can be executed at varying speeds (tempo and/or velocity); proprioceptive abilities, from a stable surface (wall or floor) to an unstable surface (Swiss ball); or planes of movement

- Learn to move within the three planes and how to integrate rotation into your movements so that your workout mimics the movements of everyday life and sport. These movements fall into three categories:

  - **Sagittal** (movements that go up and down and forward and back)

- **Frontal** (movements that go side to side)

- **Transverse** (movements that rotate the top and bottom halves of the body)

Let me explain why incorporating exercises that work on multiple planes is so crucial to achieving the strongest muscles in the least amount of time as well as the best overall fitness. Most exercise equipment is designed to strengthen one or two muscle groups at a time on a singular plane, and most current popular workouts restrict movement to a singular plane as well. This is true of the quad bench, biceps curl, hip abduction, hamstring curl, calf raise, and the triceps press. This training approach has brainwashed the average gym member into believing that all exercises must be performed in strict planes of movement, which usually tend to be the sagittal and frontal planes. Now look at the functional activities of life and sport: bending, chopping, carrying, walking, skipping, twisting, running, jumping, hopping, catching, throwing, kicking, climbing, squatting, pushing, and pulling. These activities, by their very nature, require motion in all three planes simultaneously, so that multiplane movement dominates daily life and sport. All of these component movements will combine to achieve a backhand at tennis, a golf swing, a header in soccer, a spike in volleyball, or paddling in kayaking. Everyday activities such as getting in and out of the car quickly, carrying laundry up and down stairs, and even sitting at a desk are going to be easier, more fluid, and, for those who experience discomfort, less painful.

General Instructions

Each exercise will include its own specific instructions and will be easy to get the hang of once you've done it a few times. However, here are some general guidelines to keep in mind as you prepare to get started.

Equipment

None of these exercises requires a lot of equipment, but you need to gather around you (whether you're at a gym or at home) the following:

Yoga mat

Towel (to roll and insert under your head for support)

BOSU trainer

Swiss ball

5- to 15-pound dumbbells (Never sacrifice completing the movement correctly for a heavier weight. The exercises will lose their full effect; there is plenty of time to work toward a heavier weight.)

You will see that many of the strength-training movements utilize several common gym machines; it matters less what machine you are using (i.e., brand name, etc.) and more that you choose a machine that best suits the exercise. For example, if the exercise calls for a lateral pull-down, you can use either a cable machine with two cables or one that offers a bar. As you get accustomed to the movements, use the photos as a guide to figure out which machine to use.

When it comes to deciding what weight to use for any of the strengtheners, it's best to start at a low weight (8 to 10 pounds) and gradually work up to heavier weights (15 to 20 pounds) with dumbbells, discs, or bars on a cable machine. It's important not to use too much weight: You will risk injuring yourself and/or not being able to maintain proper alignment while doing the movement.

Athletic Stance

You will begin many of these exercises in an athletic stance. This enables you to activate your core, empower your legs, and become centered and grounded.

1. Stand with your feet hip width apart.

2. Bend your knees slightly.

3. Tuck your bum so it's just under your hips but not so much that your pelvis juts forward.

4. Activate your core by pulling in and up from your lower abs, even as low as your pubococcygeus muscle (PC muscle).

Movement Groups and Progressions

Each of the five groups contains three distinct exercises building from A to B to C, with each exercise progressing and increasing in complexity, intensity, and level of difficulty. Do not try a harder progression without mastering the lower progressions. Since it takes elite athletes about four weeks to master an exercise, I am recommending that you stick with one five-movement progression for five weeks before moving on to the next.

For example, if you decide to strength-train three days a week (Monday, Wednesday, and Friday), then you would do all the A movements three days a week for at least five weeks, then move on to the B movements for five weeks, then the C movements for five weeks. You will find these programs laid out in five-week blocks in chapter 8.

Reps and Sets

For each strength-training movement, you will perform a certain number of repetitions, or reps, a certain number of times to create a set. Andy suggests doing 5 sets of 5 reps of each movement. For example, when you do 1 set of squats, you will squat and stand five times (5 reps), pause for a minute, then do another set of 5 reps. Pauses between sets should be between 1 and 3 minutes.

The Exercises

GROUP 1

A. Swiss Ball Cable Rotation

This exercise enhances your rotation ability on the transverse plane only. For this exercise, you need a cable machine, such as a FreeMotion or Keiser machine, and a Swiss ball. Most people don't rotate well, and this is a good way to activate the muscles of the back, arms, and abs that enable rotation. When using any cable machine or other weight-bearing machine, begin with the lowest amount of weight and gradually increase over a couple of weeks.

1. Get into athletic stance (see page 80).

2. Wrap your arms around the Swiss ball and press it against your body. Try not to round your back over the ball.

3. Grab the cable with your right hand, staying extended through your spine.

4. Rotate toward your right arm side without moving your hips or your lower body.

5. Do 5 reps, 5 sets, and repeat on the opposite side.

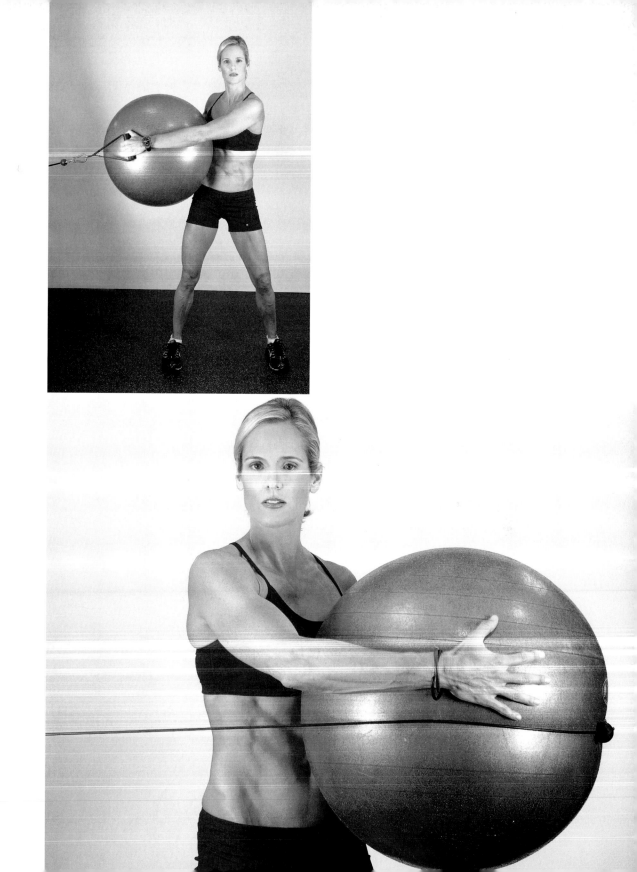

B. Fixed Medicine Ball Rotation Pass

This exercise progresses from a single plane of movement through biplanar to triplanar, as well as creating intensity. Unlike most of the movements, this one requires that you work with a partner. You will also need a wide Thera-Band loop and a medicine ball weighing 5 to 10 pounds.

1. Loop a wide Thera-Band loop around a stable surface (such as a nearby weight machine) and put the other end between your bum and your lower back.

2. Squat down and walk backward so you stretch the band to get some tension; this tension also helps to fix your lower body so it doesn't move when you pass the ball (see below).

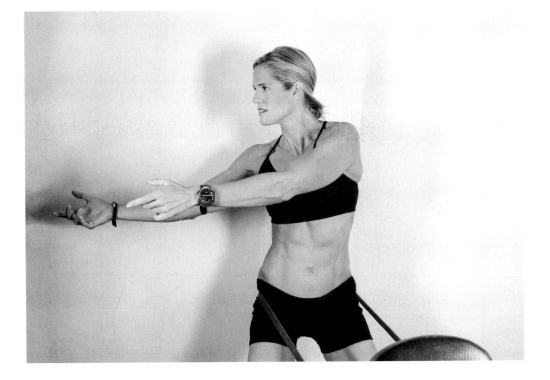

3. Have your partner stand about 3 feet away from you off to the side and throw the medicine ball so you can catch it in front of you, at belly button level.

4. As you catch the ball, rotate to the side away from your partner, absorb the weight of the ball, and then pass it back.

5. Do 5 reps, 5 sets, then have your partner switch sides, and do 5 reps, 5 sets, on your opposite side.

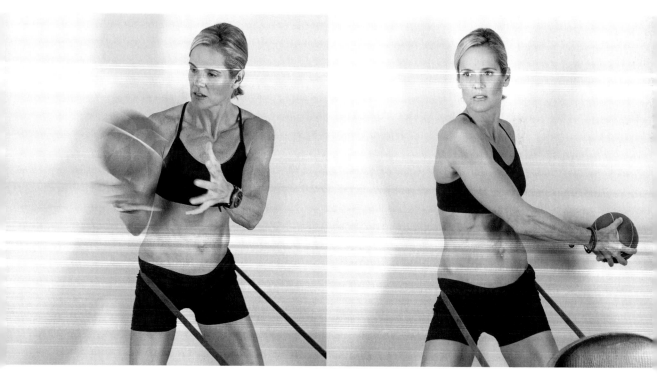

C. Alternating Cable Squat Rotation

This exercise uses a cable machine and works on both the sagittal and transverse planes. By alternating sides, you create rotation, working your core, your quads, and your arms.

1. Adjust the cable to a low position at your desired weight.

2. Stand facing the machine with your feet shoulder width apart and the cable centered between your feet, standing far enough from the machine to make the cable taut.

3. Get into a deep squat position and grab the cable with both hands.

4. Fully extend your entire body and rotate the cable up and to the right side.

5. Return to your starting position, then rotate and fully extend to the left side.

6. Do 5 reps, 5 sets.

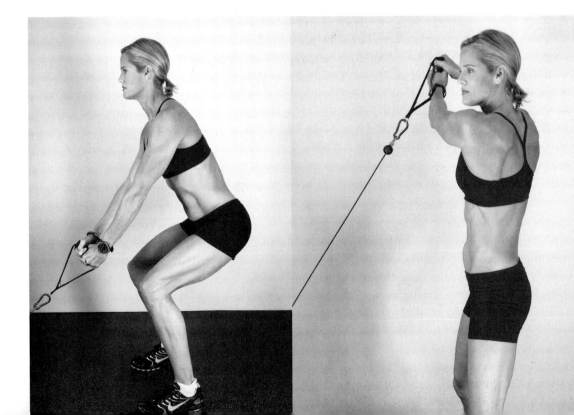

Stabilize Your Joints

Pay close attention to any cues to activate the muscles near or around your joints. Muscles move joints, so when you emphasize a certain muscle group you are essentially strengthening muscles to stabilize joints.

This progression begins on the sagittal plane, then works up to biplanar movement. It increases in intensity through the use of unstable surfaces and resistance.

A. Body-Weight Squat

This is a simple but powerful exercise that works only on the sagittal plane.

1. Begin in athletic stance (see page 80) crossing your hands over your chest.

2. Squat down, pressing your weight into your feet. Make sure that your feet are pointing straight ahead, knees over your toes. Make sure you keep your bum tucked.

3. Return to standing.

4. Do 5 reps, 5 sets. This is deceptively simple but arduous!

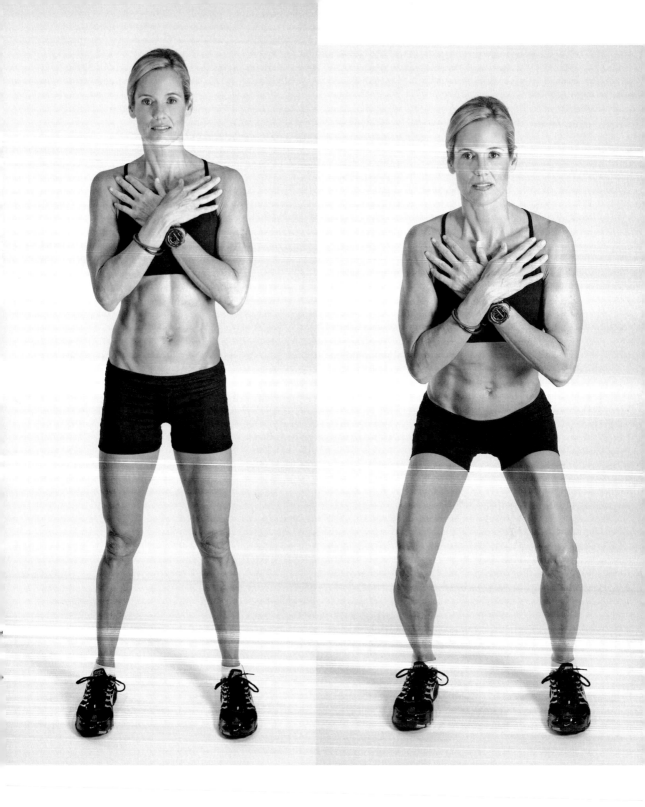

B. BOSU Dumbbell Squat

Although this exercise is similar to the movement described above, we're increasing the intensity by adding dumbbells (choose 10- to 20-pound weights) for resistance and an unstable surface (the BOSU trainer). If you don't have a BOSU trainer handy, you can use any kind of unstable surface such as a balance board or a balance mat (Airex pad).

1. Place the BOSU trainer with the flat side up. Stand on top in athletic stance (see page 80) with a dumbbell in each hand at your sides.

2. Squat down, pressing your weight into your feet, making sure that your feet are pointing straight ahead, knees over toes. Make sure you keep your bum tucked.

3. Return to upright position.

4. Do 5 reps, 5 sets.

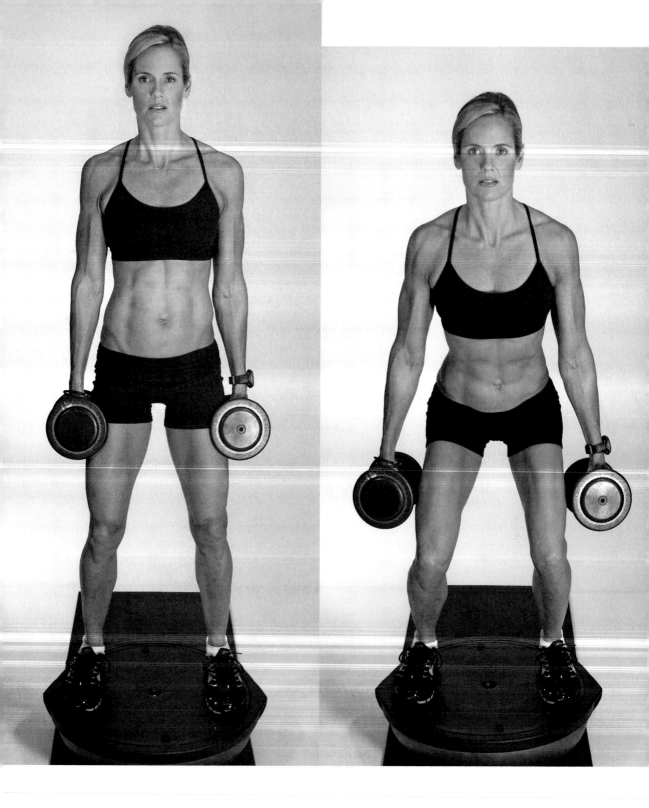

C. Rainbow with Medicine Ball or Weight

This exercise can be done standing. The photos show it seated, which is an alternative that you might find easier, especially if you have knee problems like me.
In either position, it's a triplanar strengthener.

1. Hold a medicine ball or disc weight; start in athletic stance (see page 80) or seated as pictured, making sure that your core is activated.

2. Squat down, bringing the weight to one side at your hip.

3. As you come up from the squat position, drive the weight up over your head, keeping knees, toes, and hips forward and rotating through the spine. Lower the weight to your other hip.

4. Do 5 reps, 5 sets, on alternating sides.

Note: If you increase your speed while doing the reps, you can incorporate further complexity and challenge.

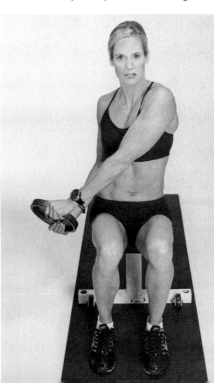

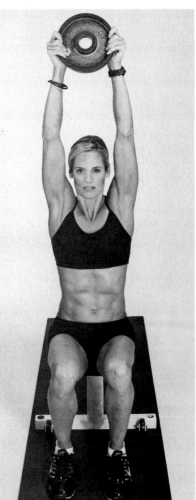

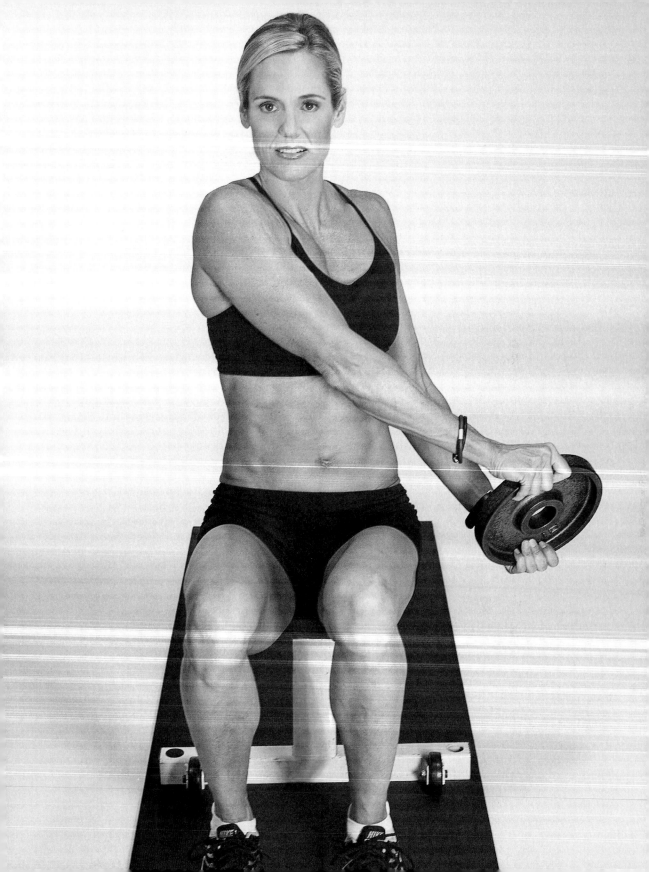

A. Dumbbell Incline Press

This exercise works on the sagittal plane only, using an incline bench.

1. Position yourself on a 45-degree incline bench with your feet straddling each side, flat on the floor. Make sure your lower back is touching the back of the bench to assure proper alignment.

2. Hold a 10- to 20-pound dumbbell in each hand.

3. Making sure your elbows stay in line with your wrists, raise the dumbbells over your head.

4. Return to start position.

5. Do 5 reps, 5 sets.

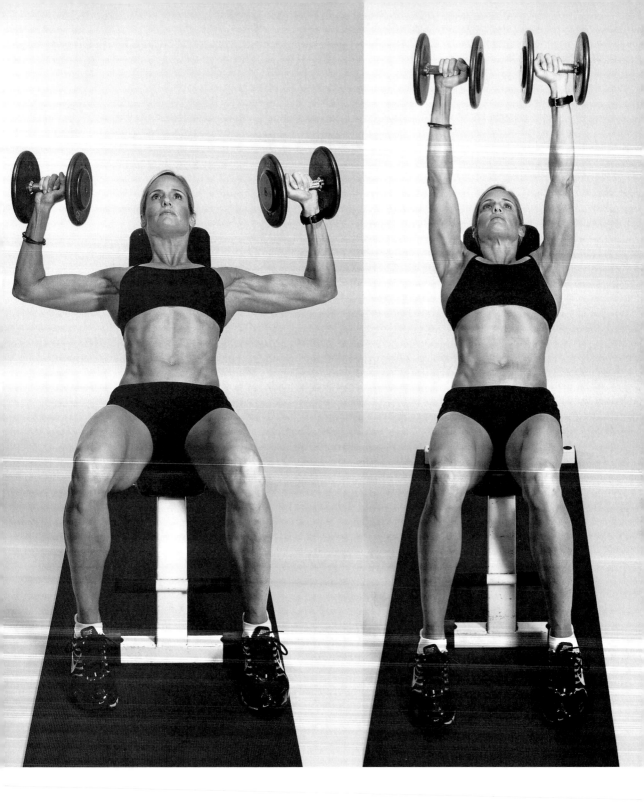

B. Smith Press Crunch

Most gyms have a Smith machine, which is equipped with an attached 7-foot Olympic bar (not seen in photo); if a Smith machine is not available, then you can use light weights or a bar without weights on a flat bench. This exercise works the sagittal plane with especially intense core activation.

1. Lie on the bench with your feet straddling each side, flat on the floor. Make sure your lower back is touching the back of the bench to assure proper alignment.

2. Grab the bar and press it up, making sure that your elbows stay in line with your wrists.

3. At the end of the press, crunch your abs just enough for your shoulder blades to lift off the bench. You are getting your core muscles to activate in conjunction with your upper body.

4. Return to start position.

5. Do 5 reps, 5 sets.

Note: If you are not working on a Smith machine or similar one, in which the bar is secured, make sure to choose a light weight that you can safely manage.

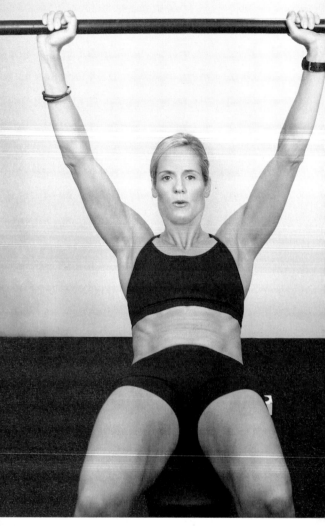

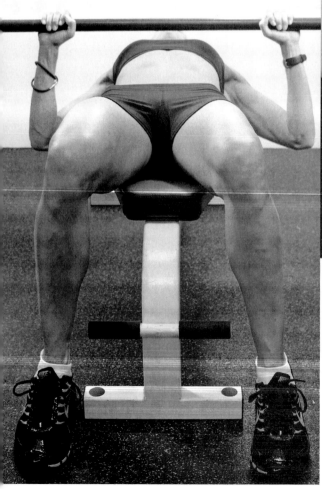

C. Bench Plyo Push-up

The plyometric goal is to produce motion as fast as possible. In this exercise, done with a bench, you will push against your body weight as quickly as you can to create intensity.

1. Put both hands on the edge of a bench.

2. Get into push-up position, with your feet a little wider than shoulder width apart.

3. Tuck your pelvis and engage your abs by pulling your belly button into your spine.

4. Lower yourself and push yourself up in plyometric fashion—at a high velocity. You will be working one plane of motion but increasing resistance. This adds progression in a different way because of the high speed.

5. Do 5 reps, 5 sets.

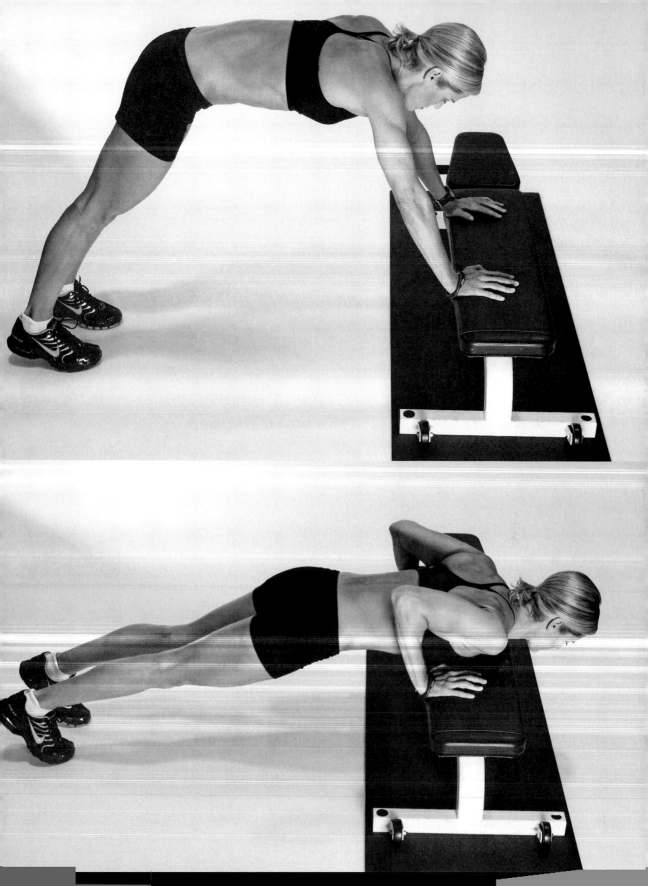

A. Ground-Based Lat Pull-down

This movement is done in a squat position on a basic cable machine to activate the lower-body power. It works only on the sagittal plane and focuses on the arms, chest, back, and core.

1. Grab the cables with each hand.

2. Take a deep-squat position and roll your shoulders back, squeezing your shoulder blades together.

3. To a count of two seconds, pull the bar or cables straight down.

4. Pause at the bottom before slowly returning to starting position.

5. Do 5 reps, 5 sets.

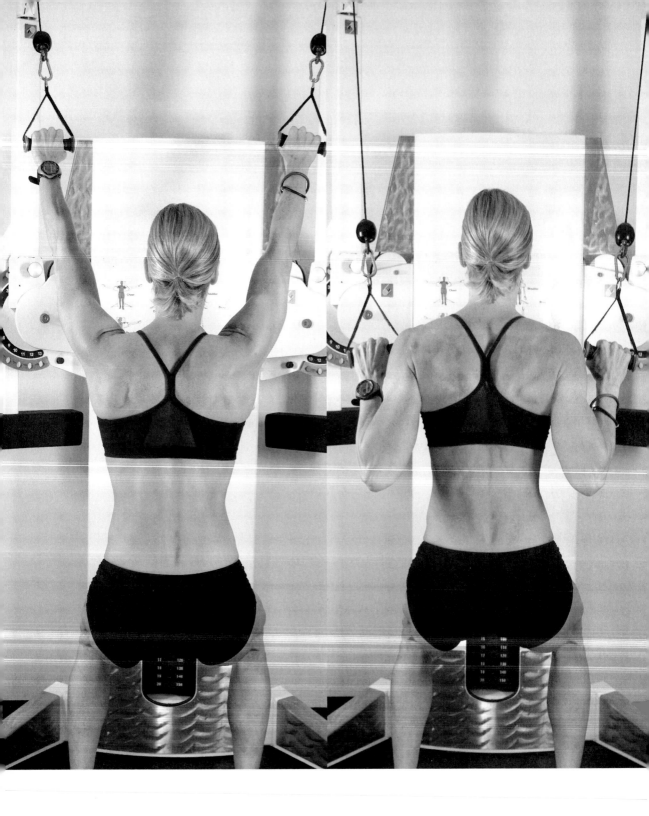

B. Single-Arm Cable Row Twist

This exercise uses a cable machine to work on both the sagittal and transverse planes.

1. Get into athletic stance (see page 80) and roll your shoulders back, squeezing your shoulder blades together.

2. Grab the cable with one hand, arm extended, and step back a bit to get some tension in the cable, then return to athletic stance or a slight squat for more intensity.

3. Pull the cable all the way back, keeping your elbow close to your body.

4. At the end of the movement, rotate your torso toward the arm you are using.

5. Do 5 reps, 5 sets, on each side.

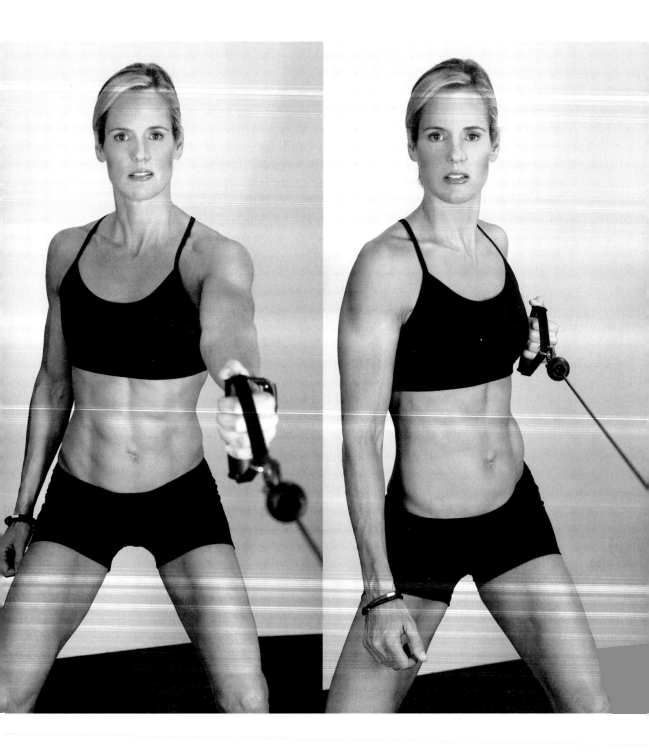

C. Cable Push-Pull Rotation

This exercise moves from a single plane through biplanar, thereby increasing muscle activation.

1. Get into a deep lunge position with your right leg in front of your left.

2. Keeping your right leg in front, use your left arm to grab the "pull" cable; with your left leg in back, use your right arm to grab the "push" cable.

3. Pull and push the cables simultaneously, rotating your torso through the exercise.

4. Do 5 reps, 5 sets, on each side.

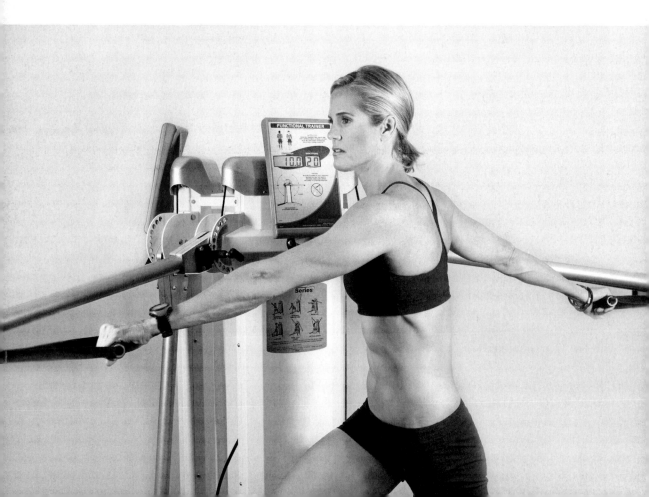

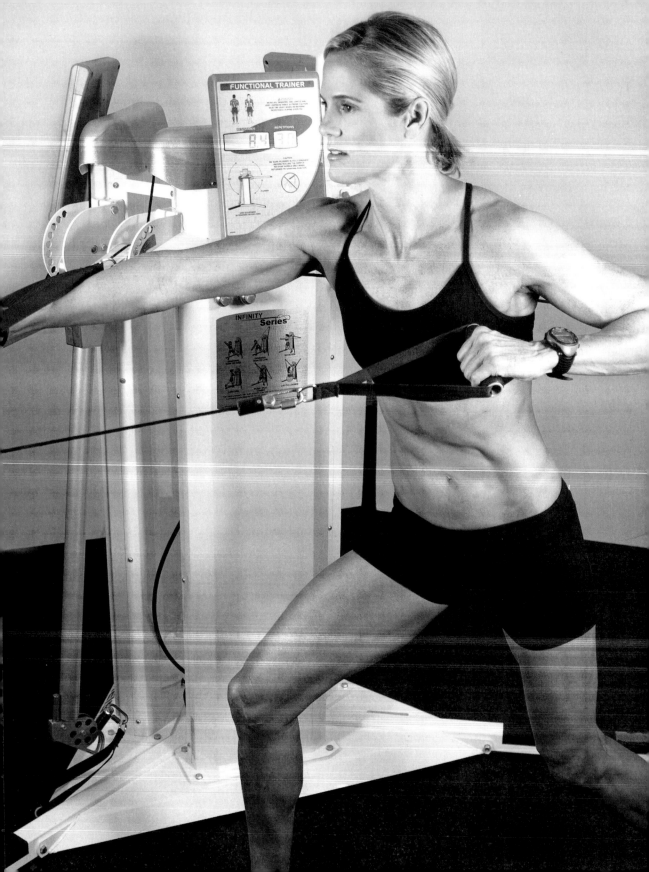

GROUP 5

A. Lateral Cable Walk-out

This exercise works on the frontal plane, strengthening the core, arms, and upper back.

1. Stand to the side of the machine in a squat position about 3 feet from the machine. Grab the cable with both hands. It should feel taut.

2. Take two steps to the right, one at a time, squatting as you step. Remember to engage your core as you descend and ascend.

3. Take two steps back.

4. Do 5 reps, 5 sets, on each side.

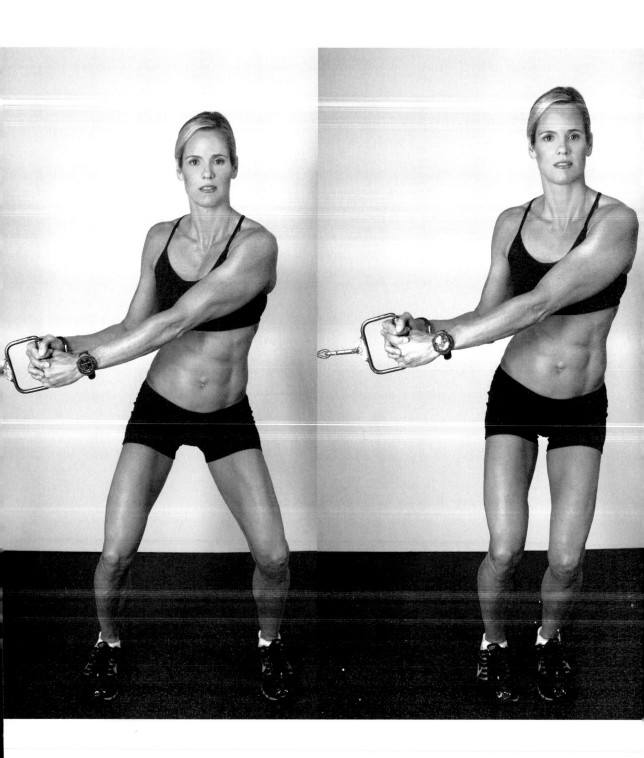

B. Side-Bridge Cable Row

This exercise works on both the frontal and sagittal planes and engages your core.

1. Assume a plank position (not shown) a few feet away from a cable machine with your body perpendicular to the cable, then turn and lean on your right arm, which should be at a 90-degree angle to your body. Stack one foot on top of the other to create more balance, and activate your core by pulling your belly button toward your spine.

2. Grab the cable with your left (free) hand.

3. Pull the cable as if you're doing a row while holding yourself still in the side plank position.

4. Do 5 reps, 5 sets, on each side.

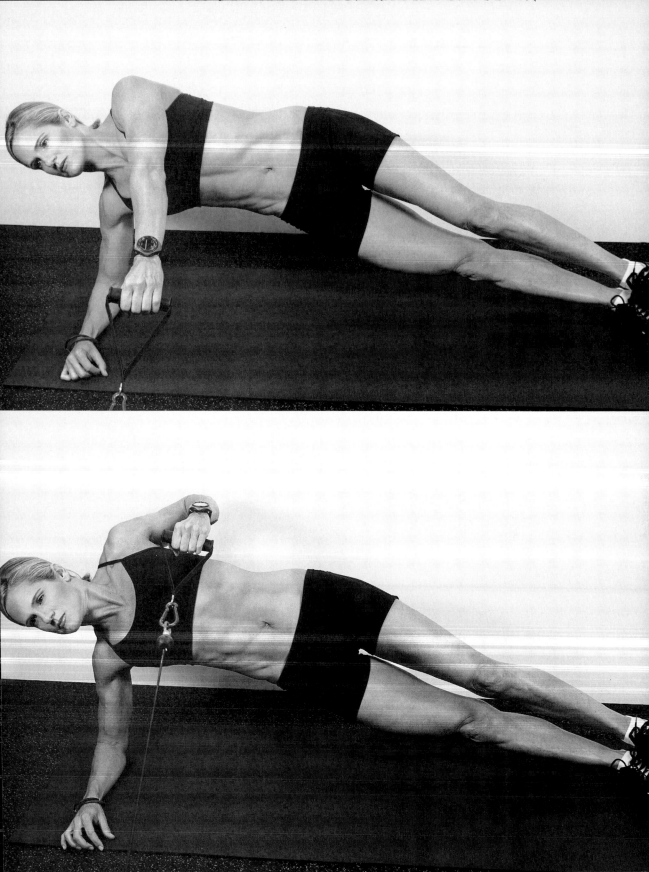

C. Star Push-up

This is a challenging exercise that you might need to work up to in its full manifestation, so please note the adjustments below. You will move on three planes of movement at high velocity.

1. Start in normal push-up position. Remember to tuck your pelvis and engage your core.

2. Lower yourself to the floor.

3. As you push yourself up, rotate your body to one side and raise your arm and leg in the air, then return to push-up position.

4. Do 5 reps, 5 sets, on each side.

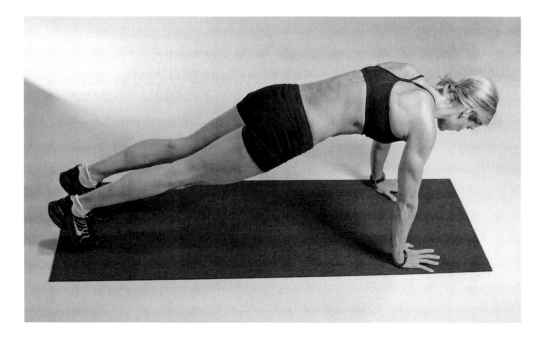

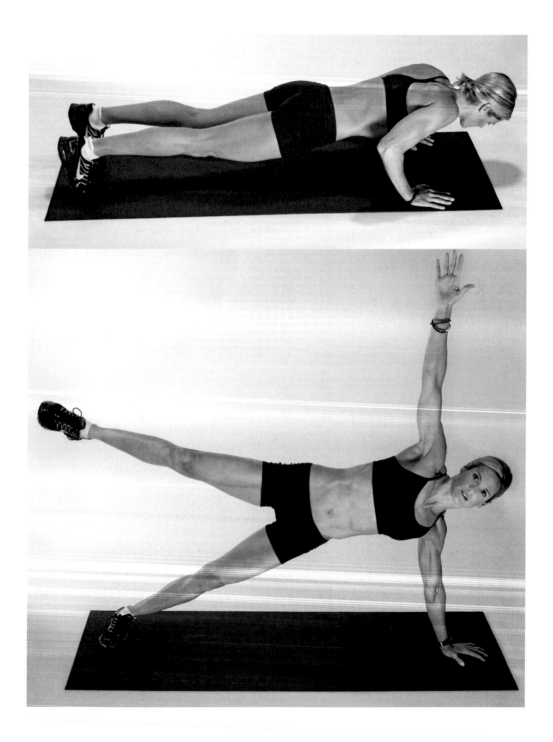

As you become more familiar with these movements, keep in mind the three key components: efficiency, progression, and dynamics. The efficiency comes with careful execution of the correct biomechanical principles of each exercise, so pay attention to the details about positioning and alignment.

Most of the exercises emphasize full range of motion for joints that are frequently moving and focus on the stabilization of the joints that move less. You want to try to make sure that movement occurs in only the joints where it is desired and that no compensation occurs in other joints. This will ensure the right muscle-activation patterns within a movement.

The progression can come in many ways. You can progress in terms of the complexity of the movement (single plane to multiple planes) or in velocity (low to high). You can create an unstable surface to work on, and you can increase the number of muscle groups/joints involved in a movement. Each of these progressions is reflected in the series. Although there are only five exercise groups here, it is important to cover all of the muscle groups and joints of the body, with an emphasis on those that are most important. When identifying your weaknesses and working to overcome your deficiencies, you might want to include more exercises that emphasize the deficiency. And when training for a specific sport, you might want to include more exercises that mimic the motions of the sport. When I work with Andy early in the season, he always begins by showing me how to overcome my deficiencies, and as I move closer to competition, he emphasizes more of my sport movements.

The dynamic component is achieved using various tempos (speed), different levels of proprioceptive abilities (working on unstable surfaces), and a variety of movements in all planes. This includes exercises that move the body through multiple planes simultaneously. Since activities in our lives and in any sport are multiplanar, dynamic exercise is just as ideal for athletes preparing for their sport-related movements as it is for nonathletes who want to improve or maintain movement in daily life.

In the next chapter, you will build on many of these principles as you begin to do the resistance stretching techniques that are another important part of your physical fitness arsenal.

5

STRETCHING
The Ki-Hara Way

|||||||||||||||||||||||||||||||||||||||||||||||||||||||||||||||||||||||||||||||||||||||||||||||||||||||||||||||||||||

When I decided to make a comeback (I've done this now three times, mind you), I knew I had to train differently. One of the first things I learned about myself was that I needed much more flexibility. What had been my routine? I'd pinwheel my arms by the edge of the pool before diving in, maybe touch my toes (or try to). That was it. When you're young and confident, especially as an athlete, you assume that you're flexible. But as we all know, one of the first signs of aging is a loss of flexibility.

Stretching is important for people at any age but especially once we pass thirty. As we age, our bodies naturally tighten up—our joints become less mobile (usually because of loss of cartilage and damage to connective tissue, causing decreased range of motion, stiffness, and inflammation), and our muscles stay in a contracted position for long periods (sitting at work, driving, watching TV), which leads them to atrophy. When your muscles atrophy they don't only lose their strength, they actually shrink and lose mass. At the same time and for the same reasons, as we age our bones lose density. However, much of this decrease in motion and strength can be avoided if not reversed through a combination of diet and strengthening, as we saw in the last two chapters. In this chapter, you will continue to build on the benefits of a good, clean diet and the strengthening exercises by practicing stretching techniques that will help to stabilize the joints as you lengthen, tone, and balance your muscles.

When you increase your range of motion you not only protect yourself against injury, you also increase your body's ability to be efficient, which translates into speed for a swimmer or runner, accuracy for a tennis player, and strength for a rower or cyclist—in other words, better performance in any sport or physical activity.

Understanding Resistance Stretching

When I was younger, I assumed that flexibility was important to a swimmer, but I didn't quite understand what this meant or how it played out both in my body and in the water. I'd never thought about how true flexibility really worked until I started doing resistance stretching. For the past several years, I've been working exclusively with Steve Sierra and Anne Tierney of Innovative Body Solutions, who have helped me achieve incredible results. Their method of stretching has literally changed my body. I've become not only faster in the pool but also more in balance with my skeleton, joints, and muscles. My body now works like a well-oiled machine.

At first not even my coach, Michael Lohberg, understood how sixteen simple movements could make such a difference in the pool. But they did, and now Michael is a total convert. The other great thing about what I do with Anne and Steve is that their training is based on the same principles used by Andy O'Brien, my strength-training coach, which means that the exercises you are about to learn build on and reinforce those you learned in the previous chapter. It's been awesome for my trainers to be in sync and to have come to similar conclusions.

Anne and Steve call their method Ki-Hara. In ancient Chinese philosophy, *ki* (sometimes called *chi* or *prana*) refers to the circulating life energy thought to be inherent in all living things; *hara* refers to the vital center of the self. The *hara* references the part of the lower abdomen and pelvis near the genital organs, located a half inch below the navel and a half inch inward toward the spine. This point also happens to be the body's central axis (its point of gravity and balancing point). Here is where your most vital source of *ki* is stored, so when you activate it, nurture it, and strengthen it, you feel its positive impact throughout your body. I can attest to this. These stretches make me feel balanced.

They will target not only those areas of your body that you are aware of needing stretching but those that you're less aware of, so you end up feeling more limber and nimble, and are able to move more fluidly. Biomechanics has shown that the best way to stretch muscles is by contracting *and* lengthening them at the same time, or eccentrically. What's the difference between concentric and eccentric training? Concentric training is most easily thought of as the muscle contraction when a weight is lifted. The muscle fibers shorten while contracting to lift the load, as in the upward movement of a biceps curl. An eccentric muscle action is when the muscle fibers lengthen to lower a load, as in the downward movement of a biceps curl. While the fibers are lengthening, they're also contracting to return the weight to the start position in a controlled manner. Eccentric training builds more muscle power, helps to create fast-twitch muscles (which I use in sprinting), and speeds recovery.

Eccentric training is one of the bases of resistance stretching. How does it make you feel? Full of energy and brimming with a tangible sense of control in your hands, your feet, and your torso. You feel especially grounded and have a keener sense of proprioception (how

Balancing Muscle Groups

Muscles across from one another through the center of the body are called balancing muscles. An example would be your central quads and hamstrings, and your central adductors and central abductors. Why does this matter? Because if your target muscle (the one being stretched) does not release its tension, then you need to stretch its balancing muscle group. It is not usually the muscle that you're trying to stretch that's limiting you but rather the balancing muscle group that you cannot shorten sufficiently to allow you to move into the stretch. Here are the balancing muscle groups:

Medial hamstring/lateral quad

Central hamstring and hip flexors/central quad

Lateral hamstring/groin

Abductors/adductors

Latissimus dorsi/deltoid

Chest (pec major and anterior delts)/back (upper traps and posterior delts)*

Chest (pec major and calves)/back (midback)**

Chest (pec minor and biceps)/back (posterior delts, traps, triceps)***

* Try an eccentric push-up (page 138) and a kneeling twist (page 140).
** Try a can opener (page 142).
*** Try a tabletop (page 148) and a Y closer (page 144).

you feel in relationship to your environment). You also feel more agile, balanced, and stable.

Steve and Anne's basic resistance-stretching approach is made up of sixteen exercises. Their technique is based on four key principles that you will execute with each movement:

1. When beginning a resistance stretch, you will always start in the contracted or shortened position. As you stretch out, you also create resistance, maintaining the intensity for the entire stretch—not just at the beginning or the end.

2. You always need to be careful not to hyperextend (or lock) any joint. Instead, keep a small bend in your knee or elbow.

3. Throughout the movement, focus on maintaining a steady contraction, remembering to keep your core tight and feel the muscles working. Keep the resistance steady, at an intensity of about a 4 or 5 out of 10—do not fight yourself too much. (This is true especially when stretching the legs because they are stronger than the arms, so you must regulate the force.)

4. Never force a stretch. If one muscle group doesn't seem to be "working" or stretching, then simply go to the balancing muscle group (see Torres Tip opposite) and work on that. Then go back to the target muscle group that was giving you trouble, and you'll notice that stretching is easier. For example, if you feel like your central hamstring is exceptionally tight (and it has adequate strength), then go after the central quads and hip flexors to begin to loosen up the hamstring.

All of these movements can be used to strengthen the muscle groups as well, by reversing the starting position. Instead of starting in a short or contracted position, start in the extended position.

Three Hamstrings

Did you know that your hamstrings are made up of three separate muscles—the central hamstring, the lateral hamstring, and the medial hamstring? In order to stretch and strengthen them adequately, you need to stretch them separately. This will stabilize your joints and help you avoid knee and hip injuries.

After practicing these sixteen movements for only a week or two, I not only felt limber and looser, I felt stronger, as if I could literally squeeze the energy from my muscles. The resistance stretches made my body feel vital and completely interconnected. As Steve explains, "Our philosophy is to create balance and efficiency in the body." I promise, after even a few days practicing these movements, you will feel your body almost bounce with life. Ki-Hara is simple and doesn't require stretching machines or elaborate and painful motions. It takes only twenty minutes to do all sixteen stretches, and they will make you stronger and more flexible—immediately.

It's important to keep in mind that each movement can also be executed as a strengthener by simply reversing the starting position. So if you want to add more strengthening to your workout (in addition to the progression movements you're doing from chapter 4), just reverse the instructions. For instance, if you want to strengthen the central hamstring after stretching it, start the same movement from an extended position, instead of a contracted position. (This will make more sense below, when you are actually doing the movements.)

You can also make these exercises more endurance-based and aerobic by doing the stretching and the strengthening exercises one after the other, continuously.

Basic Instructions

Although some of these principles seem simple and straightforward, in practice they require a lot of concentration, especially in the beginning when you are becoming accustomed to the different movements. You can do the sixteen stretches in less than twenty minutes, but be mindful of how you are doing them:

1. Do 5 to 10 repetitions of each exercise at least three times per week.

2. The resistance stretches can be done in any order or sequence, though I have presented them here in the order that is most common: legs or arms first; followed by exercises on your back, then kneeling, et cetera. However, sometimes you might want to do them in balancing muscle groups (see the list on page 118).

3. Extend the targeted muscle/limb only as far as you can *while resisting*, and once you feel you can't resist any more, then stop, return to starting position, and repeat. Holding a position without resistance or going past the point of resistance can cause the muscle to overstretch. (If your muscle starts to shake, then back off; the shaking is a sign that you've reached the end of your range.)

4. Be careful not to hyperextend (or lock) a joint—this happens when you go too far.

5. Remember that even though it is called "resistance" stretching, you do not resist too hard. Do not fight yourself. You want a 4 or 5 out of 10 for the resistance level, and you want *movement*! Take about six seconds each way for the resistance stretch and 2 to 3 seconds each way for the strength movements.

The 16 Ki-Hara Resistance-Stretching Exercises

1. Medial Hamstring: Bent-Leg Stretch

This stretch will focus on your medial (back and inside) hamstring.

1. Lie on your back with both knees bent. You can also prop up your head on a pillow, towel, or rolled mat. Bend your right knee up to your chest and then drop it out to the side so that your knee is in line with the shoulder on that side.

2. Place your left arm under your head for support (or use a pillow/towel/mat), cross your right arm in front of the knee (down middle of the body), and grab your heel. If you cannot reach your heel, use a yoga strap or hold on to your calf instead.

3. Kick your right heel down toward the glutes continuously, contracting the medial hamstring. At first you might not be able to feel this contraction, but as you become more familiar with isolating the three parts of your hamstring, you will be more attuned.

4. As you kick your heel toward your bum, use your right arm to pull up on the heel and lengthen your right leg out toward your shoulder.

5. Return to start position.

6. Do 5 to 10 reps on each side.

Note: Only lengthen your leg as far as it can resist; you never want to lock out or hyperextend your knee.

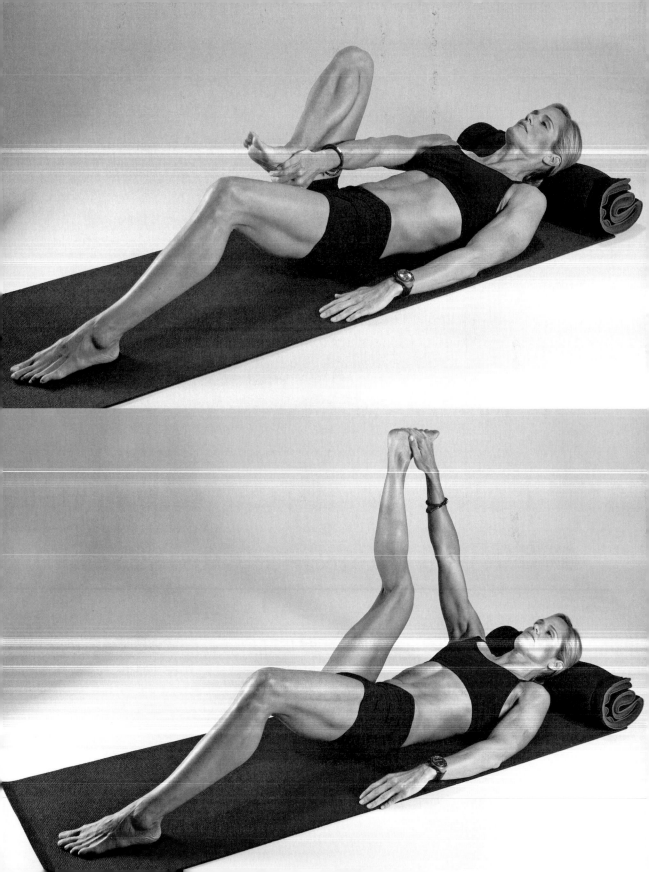

2. Central Hamstring: Bent-Leg Stretch

In this exercise you will be stretching the central hamstring.

1. Place a pillow, towel, or rolled mat under your head for support. Lie on your back with both knees bent, and bring one knee up to the chest so it is in line with your hip.

2. Use both hands to grab your heel; if this is too difficult, use only one hand. If you cannot reach your heel at all, then grab your calf or use a yoga strap.

3. Kick your heel down to the glutes, contracting the central hamstring.

4. As you kick your heel to your bum continuously, use your arms to pull up on your heel and lengthen your leg up toward your head. Only lengthen the leg as far as it can resist.

5. Return to start position.

6. Do 5 to 10 reps on each side.

Note: The knee that is bent into the chest should not move toward or away from the body. If the hip flexor starts to cramp, then move your thigh away from the body and keep it stable. Or you can go to the balancing muscle group and do the Hip-Flexor Lunge.

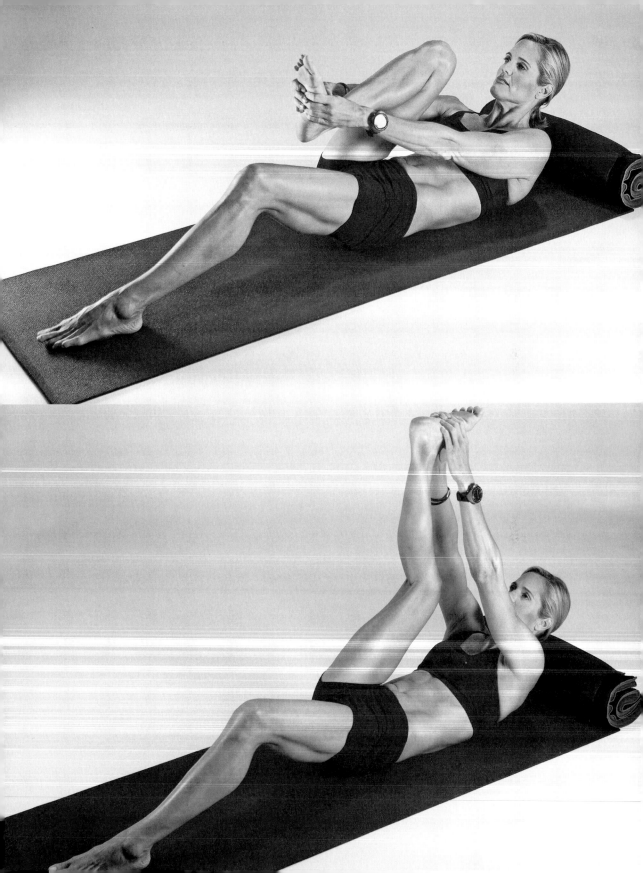

3. Lateral Hamstring: Bent-Leg Stretch

This stretch will focus on your lateral hamstring and glutes. The lateral hamstring tends to be the tightest of the three hamstring muscles, so don't be surprised if it's the most difficult to stretch.

1. Lie on your back with both knees bent.

2. Bend your right knee up to your chest and cross it over so it is pointing toward your left shoulder.

3. Use your left hand to reach across your calf (not your thigh!) and grab your right heel. Use your right arm to push on the outside of the right knee to keep it adducted across the body. Be sure you are stable and not rolling to the side of the leg on the floor. Your back should be flat against the floor, and although your hip might come off the ground slightly, you can try to minimize this by engaging your core. If you cannot reach your heel, then grab your calf or use a yoga strap.

4. Kick your right heel down toward your glutes, contracting the lateral hamstring. As you kick your heel to your bum, use your left arm to pull up on the heel and lengthen up toward your opposite shoulder. Be sure to keep your ankle in line with your knee and your knee in line with your hip. Don't torque or twist the leg at the knee.

5. Return to start position.

6. Do 5 to 10 reps on each side.

Note: Only lengthen the leg as far as it can resist, and never lock out or hyperextend the knee.

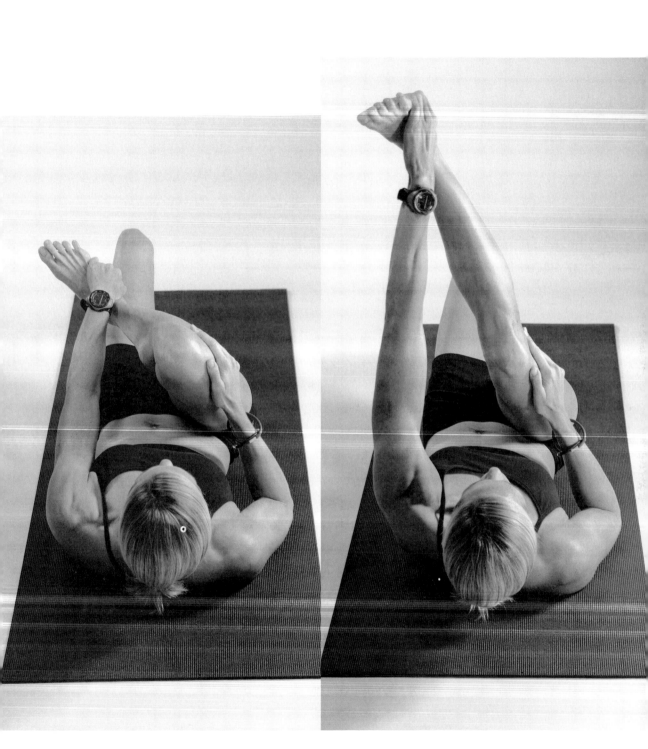

4. Quadriceps: Quad Stretch Using Swiss Ball or Wall

This stretch will focus on your quads and hip flexors.

1. Start on your hands and knees with your feet facing the wall or a Swiss ball (using the Swiss ball ups the intensity because you have to use your core and your lower leg muscles to keep balanced).

2. Lift your right leg and point your foot toward the ceiling. Move the knee 4 inches away from wall. The closer the knee is to the wall, the more difficult/intense the stretch will be.

3. Rest your toes and the top of your foot against the ball or wall. If your foot is cramping, then try to position it so it is more flexed than pointed.

4. Slowly begin to bring your left leg up into a lunge with your foot flat on the floor. Make sure that the leg is in a comfortable position and that your knee is in line with your ankle (not past your toes).

5. From here, kick your right foot into the ball/wall to contract (resist) your quads. This is like doing a leg extension at the gym.

6. As you kick into the wall/ball, use your left leg to push your body back and stretch your quads.

7. As you retract, be sure to tuck your glutes under in order to increase strength and keep proper alignment.

8. Do 5 to 10 reps.

9. Repeat on the opposite side.

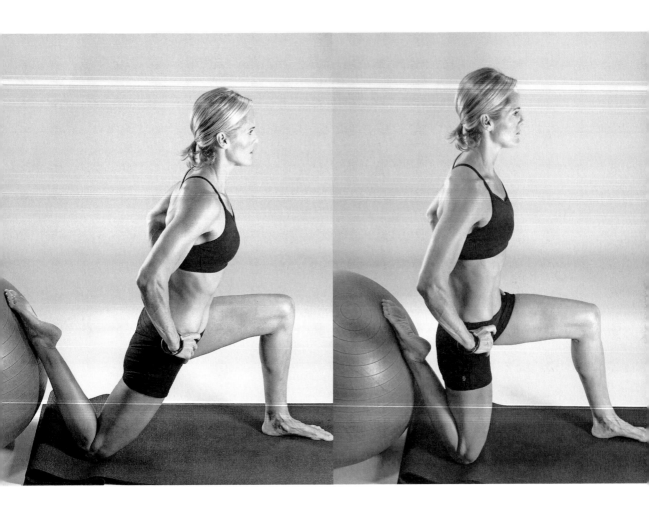

5. Inner-Thigh: Splits in the Air

This stretch will focus on the inside of your thighs (adductors). These muscles tend to be very weak because they are often neglected, so be sure to focus on the contraction or strength training in this exercise.

1. Lie on your back with your legs up in the air. Place your hands on the inside of the knees and turn your feet and thighs out.

2. Squeeze your heels together to contract (resist) the inside of the legs.

3. Continue squeezing your heels together and use your arms to pull your heels apart. Open your legs as far as they go until they cannot resist any farther.

4. Release and return to start position.

5. Do 5 to 10 reps.

Note: If your wrists hurt in this position, turn your hands so the backs of your wrists are on the insides of your knees. Also be sure to relax your shoulders.

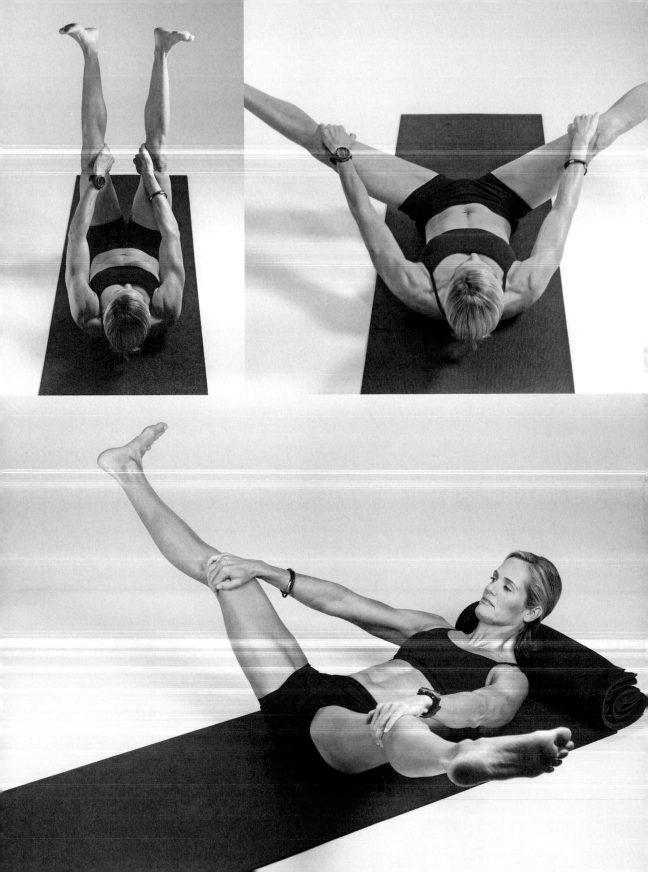

6. Outer Thigh: Knee to Chest

This stretch will focus on the outside of your thighs (abductors; iliotibial band, which stretches from the outside of your hip down the outside of your thigh, alongside the knee, and down into the calf; the tensor fascia lata, a muscle that helps abduct the thigh; and the glutes).

1. Lie on your back with your head supported by a pillow, towel, or rolled mat. Cross your left foot over your right knee. Clasp your hands around your uncrossed (right) leg, behind the thigh.

2. Push out with your crossed left leg, contracting your glutes and iliotibial band.

3. As you contract (resist) the left leg into the right thigh, use the right leg and the arms to pull the right leg into the body.

4. Pull your right knee to your chest until you can no longer resist.

5. Release and return to start position.

6. Do 5 to 10 reps on each side.

Note: When pulling back with your arms and midback muscles, keep your neck long and don't scrunch your shoulders.

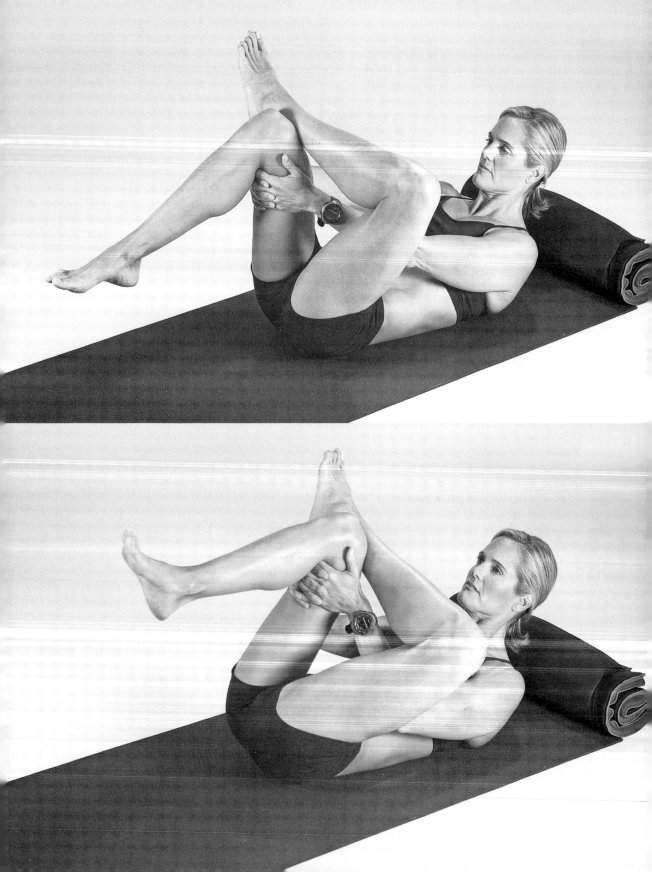

7. Groin: Butterfly

This stretch will focus on the inside of your thighs (adductors).

1. Sit on the floor with your legs bent and your heels together as close to your glutes as possible.

2. Place your hands or elbows on the inside of your knees.

3. Squeeze your knees together and use your hands or elbows to resist, then open your legs out to the sides.

4. Try to open your knees not just down, but away. This will help create traction in order to give you the best stretch.

5. Release and return to start position.

6. Do 5 to 10 reps.

Note: Never force your groin or adductors to open. Tightness in this area is usually due to the balancing muscle not being able to shorten—due to tightness, lack of strength, or injury. In this case, the balancing muscle group is the lateral hamstring.

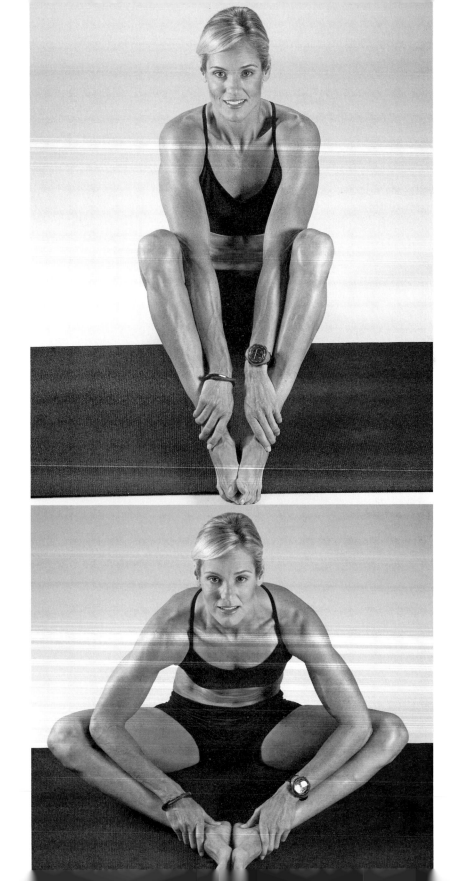

8. Hip-Flexor: Lunge

This exercise focuses on your hip flexors (iliopsoas). These muscles are often tight and weak from sitting a lot and lack of use, so both strength and stretch will be very important. They are often the cause of back problems.

1. Start in a kneeling position on the floor with your shoulders stacked on top of your hips and your bum lifted off the backs of your calves. Place your left leg in front of you with your foot flat on the floor, creating a 90-degree angle with your knee.

2. Contract your right hip flexor and quad by creating the feeling of pulling your right knee into your chest and kicking your lower leg into the floor.

3. As you do this, use your left leg to balance and pull your body forward, keeping your chest up, core activated, and body as aligned as possible so your hips are in line with the head. You are not leaning forward.

4. Release and repeat 8 to 10 times. Don't forget to breathe.

5. Repeat on the opposite side.

Note: It's very important to press the lower leg into the mat in order to generate the best contraction. If your foot cramps, try putting a rolled mat or towel under the ankle of the leg that is on the floor.

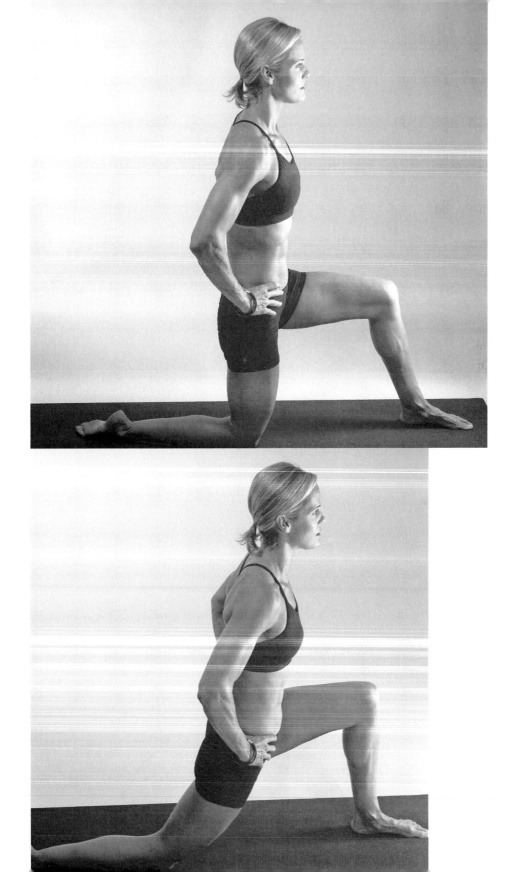

9. Chest and Biceps: Eccentric Push-up

This push-up is eccentric because you are focusing on slowly lowering to the ground. Do this stretch more slowly than a regular push-up so you can feel the stretch across your chest.

1. Start in a push-up position with your hands shoulder width apart and your toes on the floor. For a beginner version, bend your legs and do the push-up from your knees. For a more advanced version, elevate your hands on yoga blocks so that you can lower the body below the plane of the floor (not pictured).

2. Slowly lower your chest to the ground with your head up, making sure that your elbows are in tight at your sides, parallel to your body (and not sticking out), and that you maintain an external rotation of your arms.

3. Return to push-up position.

4. Do 5 to 10 reps.

Note: Throughout this exercise, be sure to keep the body flat like a plank. In order to do this you will need to activate your core by pulling your belly button in toward your spine. Be very careful not to let the belly sag by keeping your core and glutes activated—this puts unnecessary pressure on the lower back.

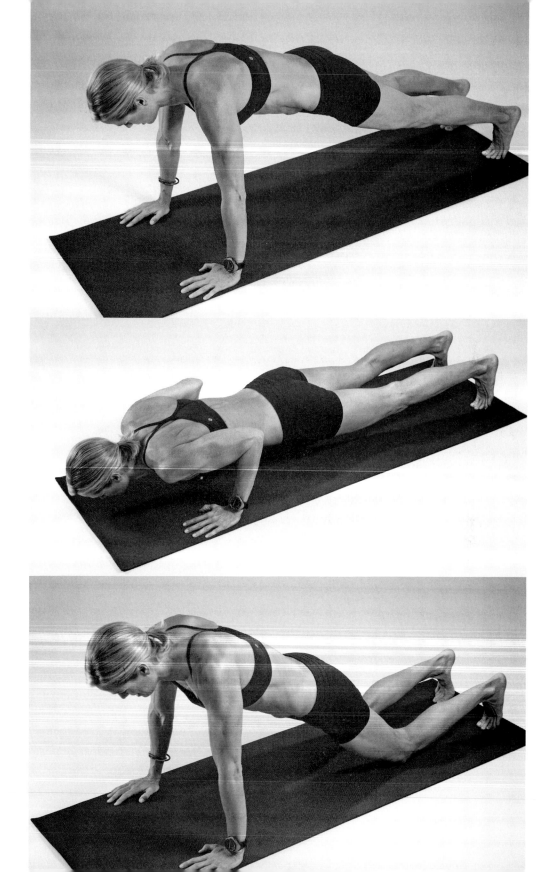

10. Trapezius and Shoulders: Kneeling Twist

This stretch focuses on your back and shoulders (trapezius and deltoid muscles) and the external rotators of your back.

1. Start in a kneeling lunge position with your left leg in front and your legs far enough apart so that you are stable. Make sure your left knee is in line with your ankle and not over your toes.

2. Place the right elbow on the left knee, at a 90-degree angle, leaving space between the armpit and knee (your upper body is not resting on your thigh).

3. Push the elbow and knee against each other isometrically to keep the body stable.

4. Keeping the right arm bent in order not to create torque in the elbow, place your left hand against your right wrist.

5. You are making a backhand motion with the right arm, pushing the back of the hand away from the body. In order to stretch the muscles on the back and shoulder, pull the left hand toward the hips while resisting with the right hand.

6. Do 5 to 10 reps on each side.

Adjustment: To add back stretch, turn the head and torso to look up at the ceiling (over the left shoulder in picture) as you bring the hand toward the hips.

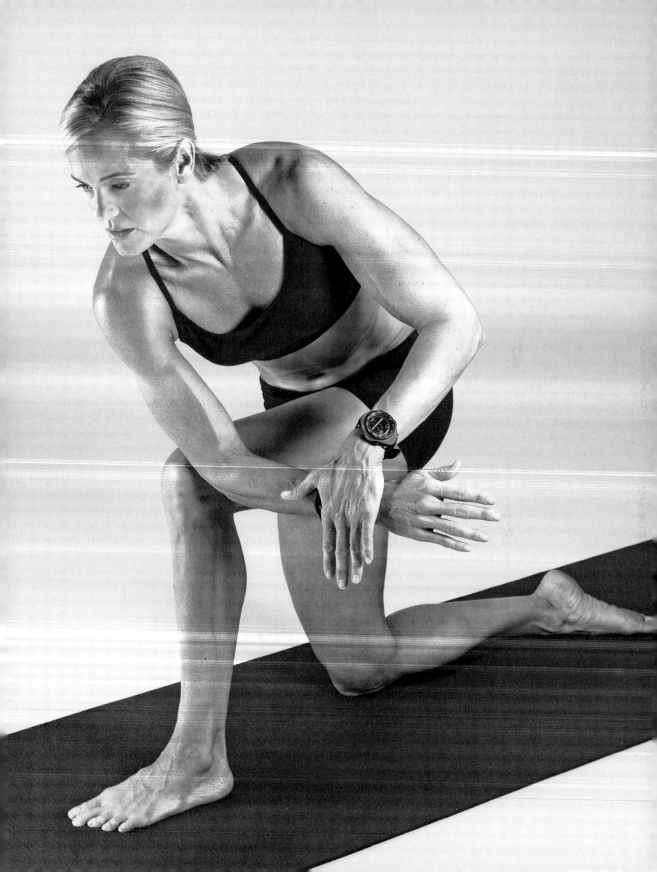

11. Back and Shoulders #1: Can Opener

This stretch focuses on the shoulders and traps.

1. Stand with your feet shoulder width apart, hands clasped (fingers interlaced) just above forehead height. Make sure the arms are bent 90 degrees and the elbows are around chin level and open.

2. Push your palms against each other and squeeze the elbows in, as if you were trying to pop a balloon between them. Be sure to keep your shoulders down and your neck as long as possible.

3. Return to start position.

4. Do 5 to 10 reps.

You should feel the stretch across the upper back above the shoulder blades and in the rear deltoid area and traps.

Adjustments:

- You can do this standing, kneeling, or sitting.

- In order to grab different muscles, you can raise your hands up a half inch at a time as you stretch.

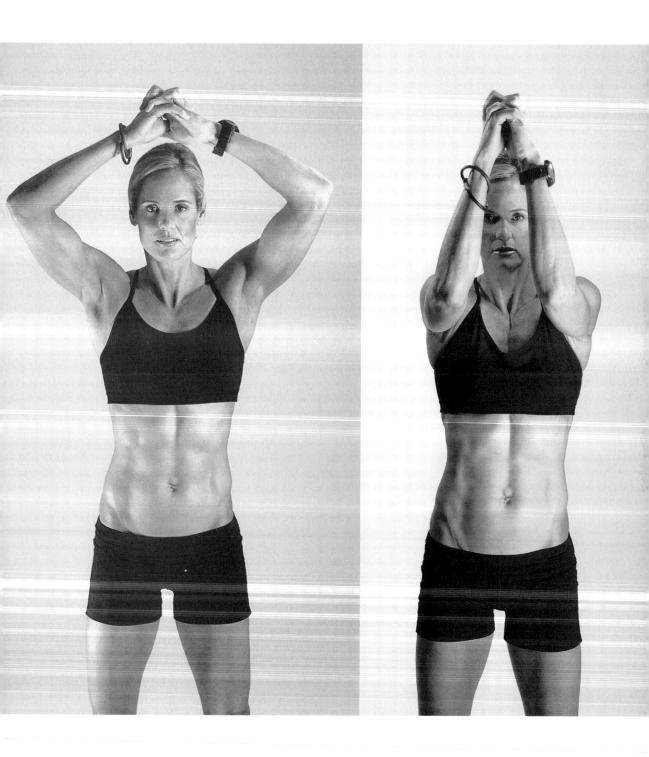

12. Back and Shoulders #2:
Y Closer

You can do this exercise sitting, kneeling, or standing.

1. Raise your left arm up at a 45-degree angle, like half a Y.

2. Place your right hand just above your wrist on the outside of the forearm.

3. Press the left arm into right hand, resisting with the right hand.

4. Continue resisting as you use your right arm to pull the left arm down and across the body toward your right hip. As you bring down the left arm, be sure to provide some lift or traction to the muscle by gently pulling the arm out and away from the body.

5. Return to start position.

6. Do 5 to 10 reps on each side.

Note: Be sure not to rotate the torso to achieve the stretch or movement. Keep the body facing forward, and focus on activating the back muscles. The core should remain engaged the entire time.

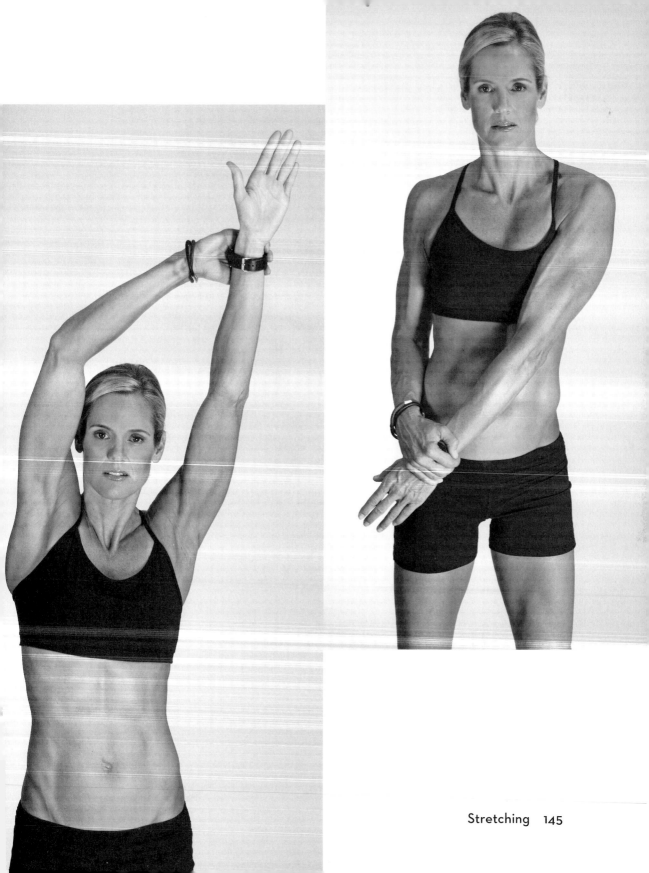

13. Lats, Obliques, and Lower Back: Kneeling Lat Stretch

This stretch will focus on the triceps, lats, obliques, and lower back (QL, or quadratus lumborum) muscles.

1. To begin, kneel on the ground with your bum on your heels. (If this position is difficult for you, then place a rolled mat or towel between your glutes and calves or sit in a chair.)

2. Place your left arm behind your head as if to scratch your back. Then place your right hand on your left elbow as if you were doing a traditional triceps stretch.

3. Contract your left elbow into your right hand as if you are trying to pull the left elbow down toward your hip. Use your right hand to pull in the other direction. Contract your oblique (side) and back muscles as your right hand pulls your left elbow toward your right knee. Keep your hips back over your heels so as to keep your alignment as stable as possible.

4. Return to start position.

5. Do 5 to 10 reps on each side.

Note: This stretch is a difficult one to get out of, so the best way is to strength-train out of it. Keep contracting your left elbow into your right hand, and instead of the right arm pulling you down to your right knee, allow the left obliques and lats to *pull* your body back up. It's a great core workout!

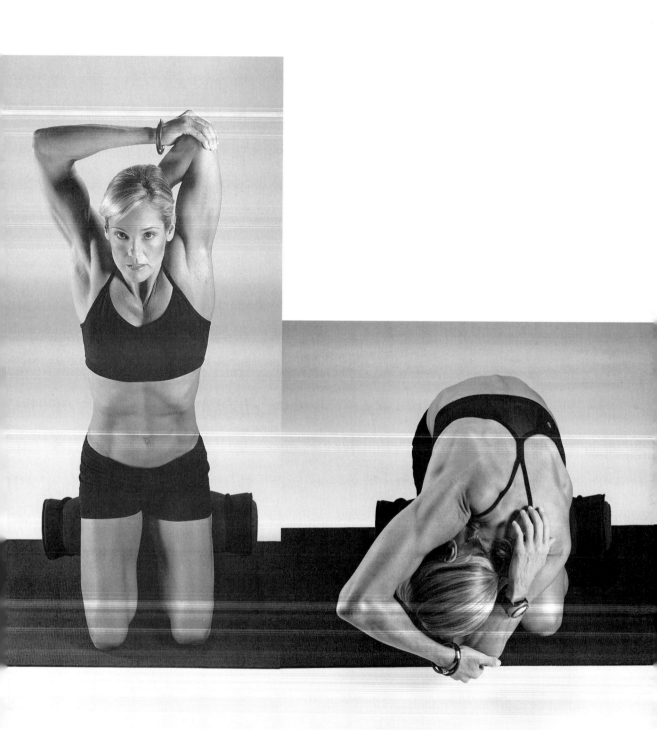

14. Chest and Forearms: Tabletop

This stretch focuses on your chest, forearms, and biceps while also working the quadriceps and gluteal muscles and passively stretching the hip flexors.

1. Start seated on the floor with knees bent in front of you, feet on the floor and shoulder width apart, and arms behind you, palms on the floor, with fingers pointed toward feet or head (toward the head is easier).

2. Pop up so that your body makes a table, keeping your knees in line with your ankles. Make sure you fire your glutes and hamstrings to pop up, and avoid locking your elbows.

3. With your core tight, try to externally rotate your upper arms (turning them out) in order to increase the stretch across the chest and arms.

4. Return to start position.

5. Do 5 to 10 reps.

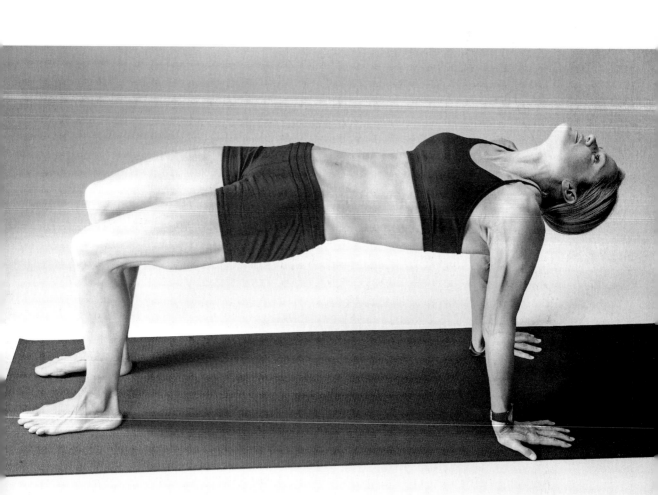

15. Trapezius, Deltoids, and Neck: Delt Closer

This stretch can be done seated, standing, or kneeling.

1. Start with your left arm bent at a 90-degree angle and your right hand on your left forearm, just below the elbow.

2. Contract the left arm up as if you are doing a side delt raise at the gym. Use the right hand to push the left arm down to the side. Be sure to give "lift" or traction by gently pulling the left arm out as you lower it.

3. Return to start position.

4. Do 5 to 10 reps on each side.

Bonus: If you tilt your head so that your right ear is by your right shoulder while doing this stretch, you will get a great neck stretch.

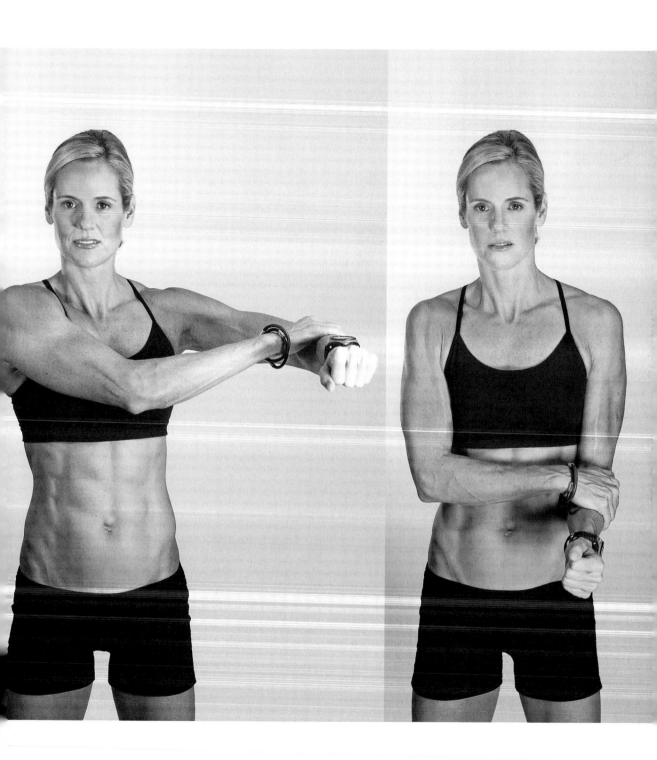

16. Chest and Calves: Elephant

This stretch will focus on your chest, calves, and hamstrings.

1. Kneel on the floor with your knees shoulder width apart and your hands palms down beneath your shoulders.

2. Pop up so that you are in a V (like a downward dog in yoga), making sure that your hands and feet are both shoulder width apart.

3. Start with your shoulders in line with or slightly ahead of your wrists. From here, use your hands to push you back onto your heels, stretching your calves.

4. Leaving your hands where they are, bring your head toward your chest to get a chest stretch.

5. Return to start position.

6. Do 5 to 10 reps.

Adjustment: If the pose is too intense on your calves or wrists, use yoga blocks under your hands. Keep a slight bend in your knees to avoid hyperextending them.

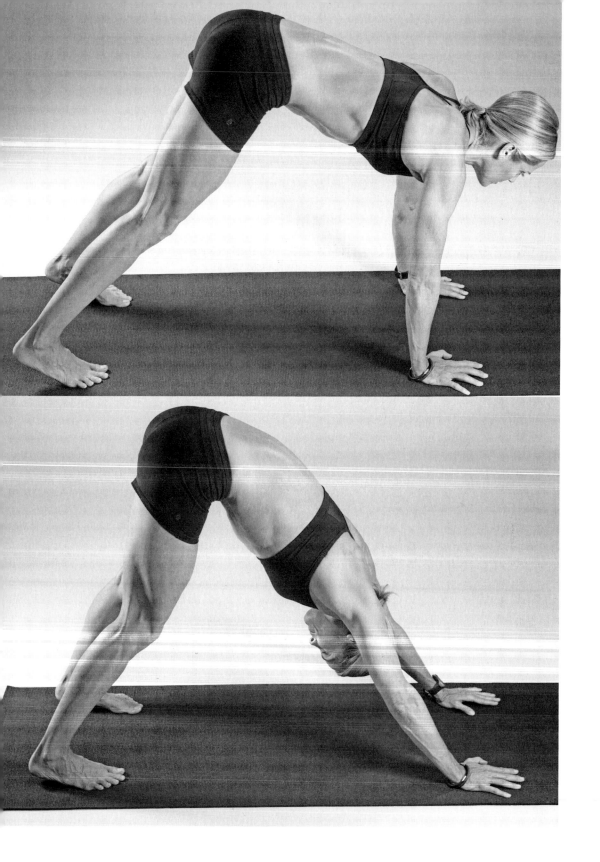

Dara's Favorite: QL-Core Twist

This stretch focuses on the lats, obliques, and lower back, via the QL (quadratus lumborum) muscle. The position may be difficult to get into, but try to work your way up to it. If you have a hard time reaching your foot, grab your ankle or calf. Also, most people rotate their shoulder only; it's best to try to incorporate the core as well, by rotating the rib cage (to get the mid-thoracic spire). Otherwise you just torque your body.

1. Sit on the floor with your right leg bent, heel toward your crotch. Take your left leg out at about 45 degrees, bending your knee slightly so it's about 4 to 5 inches off the floor.

2. Drop your left arm down toward the inside of your left leg, trying to get your shoulder as close to the knee as possible. Keep your arm externally rotated (thumbs up), and grab your toes, ankle, or calf (whatever you can).

3. Place your right hand behind your head as if you're hanging out at the beach. Contract your body forward in a side oblique twist, and try to get your right elbow to touch the ground.

4. Push your left arm/shoulder against your left knee and your left knee against your arm (so your leg stays straight up and doesn't rotate outward), and open your body up toward the ceiling.

5. Return to start position.

6. Do 5 to 10 reps on each side.

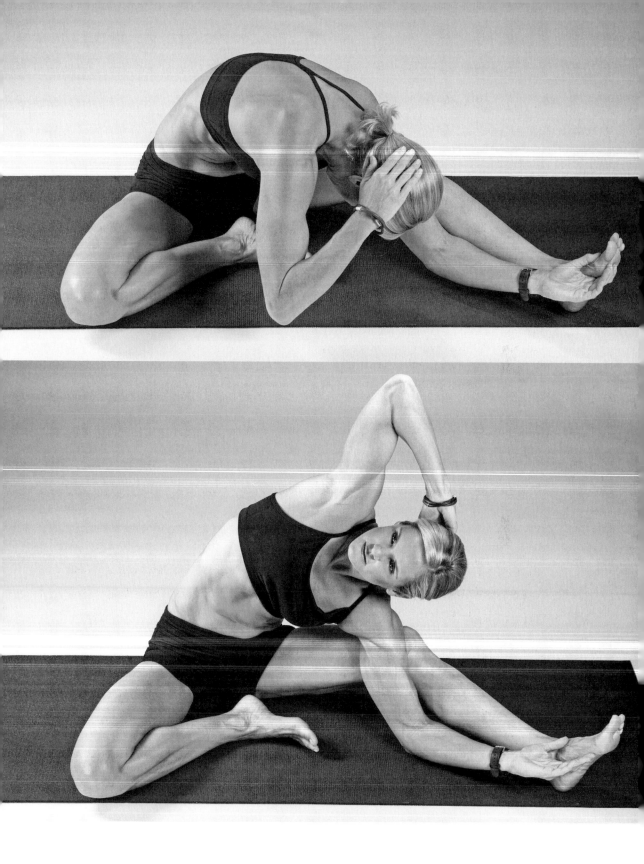

Problem-Solve Your Body

The best thing about Ki-Hara is that it's not just about stretching and strength training—it's about *solutions* for the body. That's why Anne and Steve say that Ki-Hara "unlocks greatness." Try these two simple exercises to see how easy it can be to problem-solve your body and be your own fitness expert.

A simple exercise that many people use to judge how flexible they are is the traditional standing toe touch—everyone wants to touch the ground, right? And when they can't, what do they say? "My hamstrings are tight." Well, what if we told you that without even addressing the hamstrings you could go a couple of inches farther or even *touch the ground*—in less than five minutes?

Try this: Do exercise 4 for the legs—Quads at the Wall—both strength and stretch versions—4 to 7 repetitions on each side. And if you're feeling so inclined, you can also "foam-roll" the quads (see page 190)—just about 45 seconds each side.

Now go back to the dreaded toe touch.

Better? Can you reach farther? Is there less tension in the back and the hamstrings?

Amazing, right? It's simple. Sometimes it's not about the hamstrings lengthening at all but about the *front* of the legs (mainly the quads and hip flexors—balancing muscle groups) being able to *shorten* to *pull* you forward into the toe touch. So by doing exercise 4 you just strengthened and stretched your quads so that they could *contract* (shorten) better to pull you forward into a toe touch! And if you foam-rolled them too . . . well, then you just helped to loosen them up and get some knots out of the way so that the muscles could contract better.

Do you find that your quads are extremely tight? Try this.

Start by doing stretch 4 (Quadriceps Stretch) to get an idea of what it feels like and to see how far your heel is from your glutes at the end of the stretch. Do 4 to 7 repetitions on each side.

Next, stretch the balancing muscle group by doing stretch 1 (Bent-Leg Medial Hamstring). Do 4 to 7 repetitions of both stretch and strength on each side.

Now, go back to stretch 4 and notice how much easier it is to do. That's all it takes!

Moral of the story: If you are having problems in any stretch or your muscles feel really tight, go after the balancing muscle group. There's no need to force a stretch to happen or hold it for ten minutes. Nothing will change until you "unlock" what is really going on. Use Ki-Hara to find the key.

Ki-Hara has the power to integrate all your muscle groups so that you feel efficient, energized, and strong. Because your muscle power comes from a body that is now in balance, you will increase your performance, speed, and aptitude—in whatever your activity. One power weight lifter who began resistance stretching increased his squat lift by more than 150 pounds in one week! Another man, a former football player now in his forties, lost more than thirty pounds in two months of resistance stretching (with some dietary changes, too, of course). Anything is possible!

6

CARDIO
Why You've Got to Move

||||||||||||||||||||||||||||||||||||||||||||||||||||||||||||||||||||||||||||||||||||||||||||||||||||||

like to swim fast. In fact, I like to do everything fast—I drive fast, I eat fast, I move through my day fast. But even if you're not after speed or don't think of your life as one long race, integrating a regular cardio workout into your weekly routine is a must. It's been proven again and again by scientists, researchers, and athletes themselves that the more aerobically fit you are, the healthier you are. Your cardiovascular system is a huge determinant of your overall fitness *and* your health. Obviously, the better our bodies can move oxygen through our blood, the more able we are to move efficiently, quickly, and fluidly. We think more clearly and have more energy for all the tasks of our lives.

One woman at one of my talks, a former elite-level rower, told me it took her ten years to start moving again. As Laura said:

I got up at 5:00 A.M. and trained for twenty years of my life. I would row for three hours, lift, row again on a rowing machine, eat, sleep, and row some more. My whole life was about practicing, training, and competing. Then one day while I was rowing on the Charles River in Boston, I realized I was actually looking at the trees and the people walking by. I knew I was done. I have never rowed since. Over the next ten years I didn't really do anything. Sometimes I'd run. I tried yoga and stopped. Nothing worked for me. But when I turned forty, I just hated feeling like a slug. I knew that the lack of energy I was feeling was directly related to the lack of physical activity in my life. So I joined a gym. I'm not a gym rat, but this place offers really cool classes—BodyPump, spin, and other ways of merging cardio with strength training. I finally feel like myself again!

This chapter is all about how to incorporate cardio into your weekly workout regimen and improve your approach to aerobic fitness. Maybe you'll want to try such activities as swimming, walking/running, hiking, biking/cycling/spin classes, tennis/squash, and other sports—all of which improve your cardiovascular fitness. Perhaps you'll decide to start moving with fast-paced walks through your neighborhood or around a track, start swimming, or join a gym to work out on the elliptical machine. The point is, you won't be bored, you won't dread getting exercise, and you might actually realize that moving fast—or slow—is fun!

Rating of Perceived Exertion

Regardless of our level of fitness or experience, we all need to keep track of the intensity of our aerobic workout. The simplest way to know our heart rate while working is by measuring it, but it's not likely that most of us will stop in the middle of a workout or remember to do so. One of the trainers I've worked with taught me a method of monitoring my exertion rate (i.e., how hard my heart is pumping) that is really quite easy to get the hang of once you start paying attention to your body. This is a great way to know when to back off and when to push yourself a bit harder to increase the intensity of your workout. Of course, the harder you work your body, the more fit you become and the better you will look and feel.

The method uses the rating of perceived exertion scale (also known as the Borg perceived exertion scale), a ten-point continuum based on how you experience your heart rate as you work out.

1. **Very easy.** You feel no effort and are hardly focused on the workout. You can talk while walking or jogging, for example.

2. **Moderately easy.** This is how you feel when moving about your day—doing laundry, washing the dishes, et cetera. You can talk, but you are slightly more focused on the task at hand.

3. **Easy.** This is how you feel when walking a city block or if you walk from a parking spot to the entrance of the mall. Your attention is directed and you tend to exert yourself a bit more to get to your destination. Your breathing might begin to become stronger.

4. **Moderate.** This is how you feel during a brisk walk around a track or through your neighborhood with a friend. Your intention is to "take a walk," and therefore you exert yourself more. Your breathing is stronger, and you might choose to talk less because you need to inhale more deeply.

5. **Moderately challenging.** If you increase the pace of a brisk walk to a light jog, or you place the treadmill on an angle (this is something I always do when I don't feel like a run; see page 175), you have to work harder to keep up the pace and therefore push your heart to pump harder. For most of us, it's becoming a bit awkward to carry on a conversation.

6. **Challenging.** You are walking more briskly, jogging, or walking on an incline at the same pace as in level 5, but you've now been moving for at least fifteen minutes. Your breathing is deeper, and you don't feel like talking. You might feel a bit tired, but you can keep going.

7. **Slightly difficult.** You have now reached a level of vigorous exercise. You definitely feel tired and your breathing has become quite deep. You can carry on a conversation, but it takes effort and you shorten your sentences. You can feel your heart pumping hard.

8. **Difficult.** You're pushing yourself hard. Do you remember doing a 100-yard dash as a kid, or a 25-yard swim race, or sprinting from telephone pole to telephone pole while running? Your breathing is strenuous and it's difficult to carry on a conversation. Your body is working very hard. This is the place where aerobic activity, when sustained for at least twenty minutes, can burn fat and condition your heart and lungs.

9. **Very difficult.** You're working almost near your maximum. Your breathing is labored, you want to stop, and you have to push yourself to keep going. Most elite athletes train at this level.

10. **Most difficult.** This level requires all-out intensity and cannot be maintained for very long. This is an anaerobic zone. When I do a 50- or 100-meter freestyle race, I swim at this level of exertion.

Rating of perceived exertion, or RPE, is the most important measuring tool you'll use day to day in your workouts. By managing your exertion, you can burn fat and calories and build muscle more efficiently. The levels you most want to work up to and stay in are

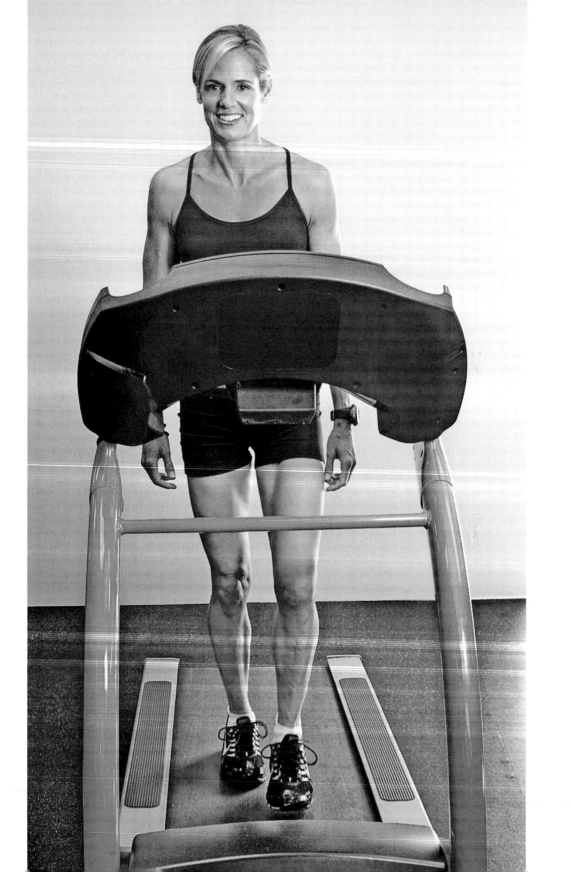

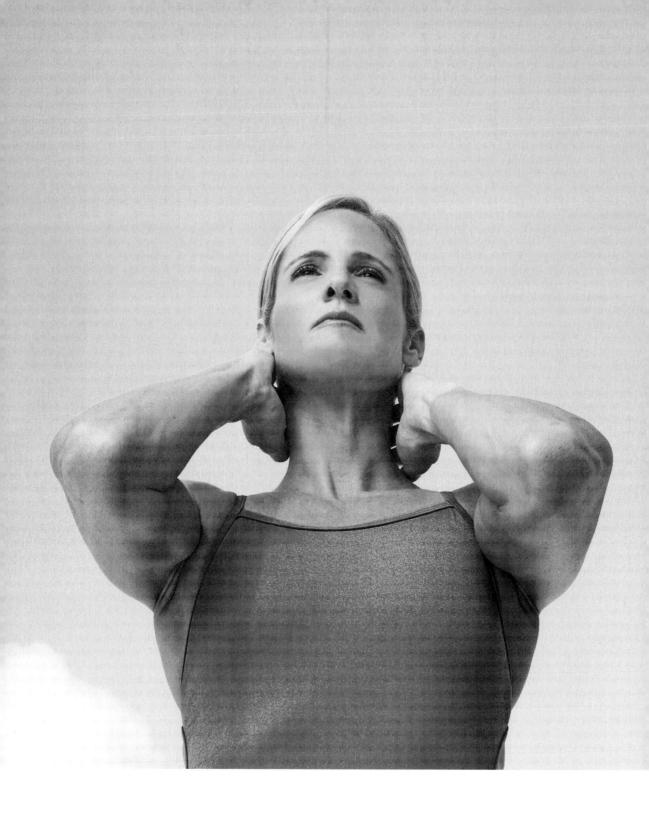

6 to 8. If you haven't exercised in a long time, build slowly from 1 to 4, knowing that in a few weeks you'll be able to warm up at level 4 or 5 and gradually hit a 6 or 7 during your workout.

For those of you who are accustomed to working out and are currently doing at least thirty-five to forty-five minutes of cardio at least three days a week, you will want to warm up at a 4 or 5 level of exertion right away, gradually building toward a 7, 8, or 9 during the course of your workout. You do not want to train at a level 10, which can be dangerous for most people except the most elite-level athletes.

Aerobic and Anaerobic Workouts

There are two cardio training zones you'll need to know about to manage your workouts for maximum benefits. Aerobic conditioning takes place when your body is working with oxygen. This type of training makes up the bulk of your cardiovascular work. The American College of Sports Medicine recommends thirty minutes of aerobic conditioning at least three to five days per week. Aerobic conditioning improves your body's ability to transport oxygen and to clear carbon dioxide. In this way it acts like an active detox, flushing impurities from your body. Aerobic conditioning also builds your endurance—so the more you sustain your heart rate over level 5, the more fit your heart becomes.

Anaerobic conditioning takes place when your body is working without oxygen because of the intensity of your exertion. Swim races over 200 meters are primarily aerobic, while shorter races are primarily anaerobic, though both short and long races require some of both. As a sprinter, I've always needed to do more high-intensity workouts and less volume. Anaerobic conditioning builds muscular power,

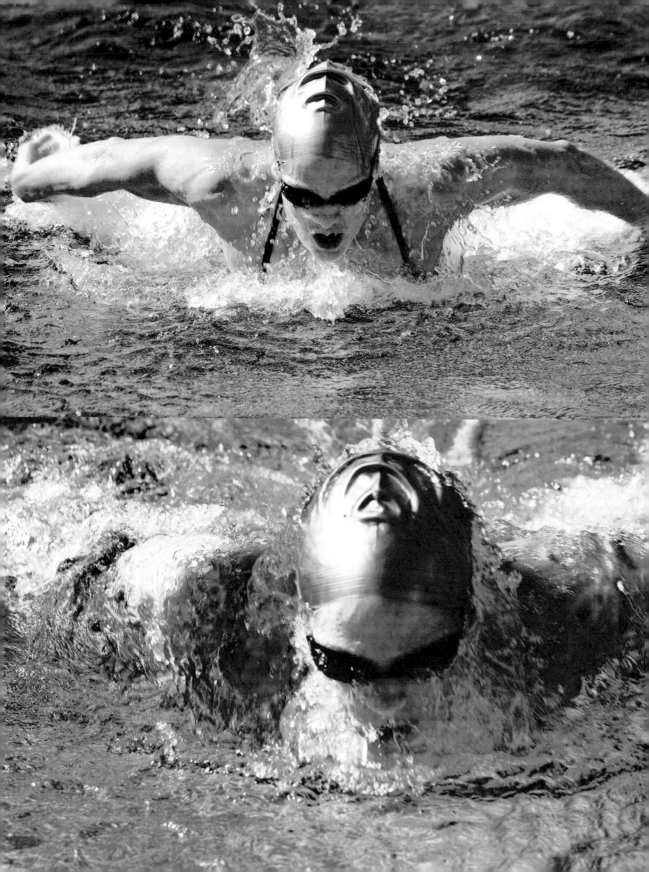

strength, and speed, all of which I rely on in a 50-meter sprint. You might not be sprinting off the blocks, but you will find that anaerobic training will become an important part of your routine. It's best to include anaerobic conditioning in your workouts only one to two times per week for general conditioning and up to two to three times per week if you are a high-performance athlete.

Cardio Activities

Getting a good cardio workout should be fun. You might already like to walk or run; or perhaps you play tennis or cycle regularly. If you're a gym-goer, you might already do run-walks on a treadmill or work out on an elliptical. If so, keep going. Cardio always increases fitness. Try to do at least thirty to forty-five minutes a minimum of twice a week, and three to five days per week to develop endurance and/or to lose weight. (See chapter 8 for specific ways to organize your strength, stretching, and cardio sequences.) Here are some great cardio activities to consider whether you want to add or try something new or are just beginning.

Swimming

Of course, I swim. I swim five times each week, for one and a half to two hours. Now, that's not for everyone. An average person could swim hard for twenty-five minutes three times a week and still benefit greatly. If you do like to swim, or want to learn, it's important to pay attention to your form so that you can maximize your upper- and lower-body strength, engage your core, keep your joints stable, and become more efficient in the water.

Socks to Swim

It might sound funny, but I wear socks under my fins when I swim. That way I'm not distracted by the soreness of my feet rubbing against the rubber and I avoid blisters.

Walking and Running

Whether you want to add walking and/or running as a form of cardio fitness to your overall workout, it's very important that you approach either exercise with good body alignment. Without it, you can develop injuries (from your neck to your spine to your hips, legs, and feet). But once you become aware of and regularly practice proper form, you not only maximize your cardio workout (by literally increasing your lung capacity), you also arm yourself against injuries, especially those having to do with your joints.

Also, I would suggest running on surfaces that give—jogging trails, the beach, a soft track, or the woods. Running can be high-impact on your knees, and an asphalt road can increase this impact, especially roads that tend to slope at the edges.

1. The first step to getting into proper body alignment is to activate your core, which entails standing with your feet hip width apart, tucking your rear enough so that your hips ride over your knees (instead of resting in a pushed-back position, increasing the angle of your lower back). Finally, contract and release your core muscles as if to awaken them.

2. Once your core is activated, rotate and adjust your shoulders so they are back, with your shoulder blades flat and down on your back.

3. From this position, look straight ahead and think of a needle and string rising from the crown of your head. With your chin straight (neither tucked nor tipped up), your shoulders back, and your core activated, you will be able to maintain a straight spine while you move forward.

When you begin moving, let your arms and wrists dangle to make sure you're not tensing or hunching your shoulders. Once you focus in on the position and state of your upper body, you can engage your arms to move with you as you walk or run.

Running is one of the oldest and most natural of human activities, but many of us think that past a certain age, it just causes too much pain—sore muscles, knee injuries, hip pain, or shin splints. When you learn how to use proper alignment to relax your shoulders, as described above, you utilize more of your core as you run, which makes you better able to stride and run with ease and fluidity.

TORRES TIP

The Benefits of Walking

Walking has been scientifically proven to be effective at

- dramatically reducing the risk of death
- lowering the risk of heart disease
- lowering blood pressure
- reducing weight
- increasing mental acuity
- improving balance
- reducing the risk of dementia
- reducing the risk of breast and other types of cancers
- relieving the symptoms of depression
- warding off diabetes
- increasing bone density
- increasing your sex drive

Now, who could resist all those benefits? And anyone can do it!

Play a Sport

If you already enjoy a sport or want to learn a new one, that's awesome. Sports have always been a part of my life, and I think they have taught me a great deal about living to the fullest. One woman I spoke to told me that she started playing competitive tennis at the age of forty-five—and has never felt better. She just loves being out there on the court testing herself, improving her game through mental strategy. As she told me, "I used to worry about not having the time to devote to it. But you know what? I made the time because playing makes me feel so good. I have two young kids, a full-time job, and I still play four to five hours of tennis every week." She feels the benefits in the rest of her life as well. "I think better, I sleep better, I feel better."

Here are some other sports that you might want to try or go back to:

Basketball: Pickup games for women in their thirties and forties are easy to find. Check out your neighborhood Y or town rec center for more info.

Cross-country skiing: This winter sport provides a great workout, usually in beautiful settings. And here's a tip: Always layer your clothing. When you start moving, you can build up a sweat really quickly, and you'll want to shed some clothes.

Rollerblading/roller-skating/ice-skating: These three activities require virtually the same kind of movement—they just take place on different surfaces. Indoor ice-skating rinks abound—regardless of where you live—and Rollerblading can be done anywhere. These are all great ways to build up your quads and glutes, too. I prefer roller-skating to blading because I feel more stable on the four wheels, but try them both out and see which you enjoy.

Biking/cycling/spinning: It doesn't require a lot to go on a bike ride. The key is finding a good course without too much traffic. Also, there are many charity rides that can get you back on the bike and help motivate you to train. Many gyms and sports clubs now offer spin classes—these are a great way to build up your cardio endurance and stamina. Cycling on a stationary spin bike at high intensity to blasting music makes the time fly and your legs burn!

Dance-inspired classes: I'm not much of the dance type, but a lot of fitness centers offer a selection of dance-inspired classes that can really kick your butt. Zumba, Nia, and hip-hop-style classes make you break a sweat and end up working your body like any kind of interval-training workout. Check one out if you like to boogie!

Hiking: For those of you who love to be outdoors, hiking is a great way to spend time in nature and get a cardio workout. You might want to invest in a pair of supportive hiking shoes, and do a bit of research on trails in your area, but otherwise, this is a pretty fast-and-easy activity to get into!

Gym Machines

I spend about half my training time in a gym. I love working out on the machines, which keep getting more and more sophisticated and varied, and in Florida, where much of the year it's too hot and humid to work out outside, gyms are my salvation. You can get a great aerobic workout in a gym setting, using the elliptical trainer, spin bike, treadmill, stepper, and other machines.

You might already work out on an elliptical or a treadmill. But here are some tips to keep in mind when using these machines:

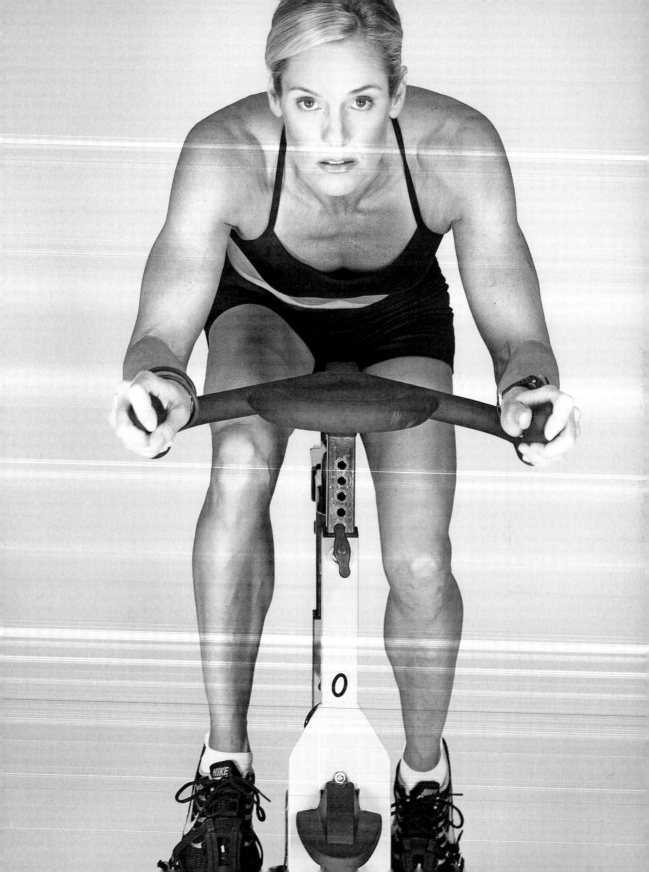

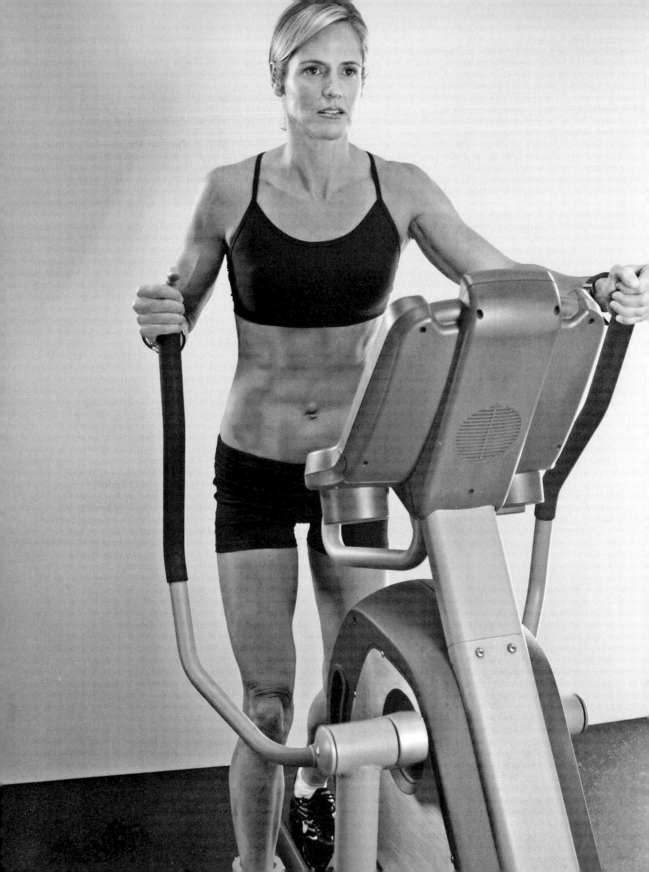

- Start on the sides of the machine, straddling the center belt of the treadmill.

- Start at low speed and gradually increase your pace.

- Utilize the incline feature on a treadmill for added resistance. This will help you target different muscle groups. For example, a low-elevation setting will target all the lower-body muscles; while a higher setting will target the thighs and glutes specifically.

- If you're new at working out on a machine, don't involve your arms too much. As you become more competent, bring your

TORRES TIP

iPod Playlist

For me, running on a treadmill or outside is much more fun when I listen to my iPod. I've shared one of my favorite playlists for you to try. Check it out!

Four Hip-hop, Four Rock

"The One," Mary J. Blige

"Empire State of Mind," Jay-Z

"Ain't I," Yung L.A.

"Single Ladies," Beyoncé

"Immigrant Song," Led Zeppelin

"I Love Rock and Roll," Joan Jett and the Blackhearts

"Sweet Emotion," Aerosmith

"Back in Black," AC/DC

arms in, close to your body. On an elliptical, you can use the handlebars to work the biceps, triceps, shoulders, chest, and back. On the treadmill, you can keep your arms moving in a forward-back motion (not side to side) to utilize more of your core.

- Keep your back straight and limber; don't bend forward.

- Keep your eyes looking straight ahead; avoid looking down.

- On the treadmill practice a good stride with front heels striking close to your body, using your back foot on the ground to help push off.

If you live in an area of the country that gets too hot or cold or wet to run or walk all year long, working out on a treadmill or elliptical is a lifesaver. Make sure you get to know the features of the machines so that you can manage your workout, going easy on some days, harder on others. And always take precautions to work out safely!

How to Approach Your Cardio Workout

What follows are some baseline tips to keep in mind, regardless of what type of cardio you do.

Start Out with a Warm-up

Whether you've been doing regular cardio workouts or you're starting again after a long pause, it's important to begin any cardio session with a 5- to 10-minute warm-up of light cardiovascular movement to increase blood flow and warm up your muscles.

If you're just starting out, you might want to simply begin walking. I trust that in a few short weeks, you'll need to jog to break a sweat—a sure indication that you've already become more fit. Whatever your starting fitness level or your age, you can—and will—improve.

If you've been working out regularly, it's still important to warm up for five to ten minutes so that you tune in to your body, give your breath a chance to circulate through it, and slowly warm up your muscles.

In the five-week plan described in chapter 8, I offer several different warm-ups to use. For cardio, a walk or slow jog is the easiest way to prep your body for the workout itself. For cycling, you should spin at light intensity for five to ten minutes.

Length of Cardio Workout

As mentioned previously, the American College of Sports Medicine recommends getting at least thirty minutes of cardio three to five times a week. You can play with these numbers, especially as you get more involved in your strength training and resistance stretching. As you learned in those respective chapters, when you increase your pace and create interval-training techniques as you do a series of exercises, you actually move your body into an aerobic zone. So if, for example, you're doing a series of strengthening or stretching exercises that lasts for thirty-five to forty minutes, you might have already accomplished thirty minutes of cardio work while strengthening or stretching.

Some of you might also like to do a cardio workout less frequently but for longer duration. Isolating certain days of the week for cardio can work for people who prefer alternating cardio with strength/stretch training. If, for example, you like to run for forty-five or sixty minutes three times a week, and do strength and stretching two days a week, then over a five-day week, you've created a good balance between strength work and aerobics. (See chapter 8 for sample workout plans.)

Hot Tips for Cardio

Here are more tips to keep in mind when approaching your cardio workout:

- The best aerobic exercise is one you love to do! So the first, most essential step of your cardio commitment is to find one, two, or three activities that you enjoy and can alternate between.

- Warm up. Warming up your muscles and joints increases blood flow and oxygen so you'll feel better while moving. The warm-up causes enzymes in muscles to burn fat faster.

- Vary activities so that you can work a lot of different muscles. Try both indoor and outdoor aerobic exercises.

- Do cardio as often as possible, while avoiding overtraining. Remember, recovery and rest from exercise are just as important as the exercise.

- Exercise for time, not distance. Don't worry about how far you run or walk; commit to twenty-five minutes, thirty minutes, forty-five—whatever works for you.

- The right time to exercise is whatever time works for you.

The more active your lifestyle, the more energy you'll have and the more calories you'll burn. Your body wants to be active—so let it! In the next chapter, you get to rest—I swear. You'll learn all about how recovery and rest are essential to staying in shape, avoiding injury, and pushing your longevity to the max.

7

RECOVERY

The Key to Your Performance

|||||||||||||||||||||||||||||||||||||||||||||||||||||||||||||||||||||||||||||||||||||||||||||||||||||||||||||||||||||||||||||||||||||||||

W hen I was younger, I associated the concept of rest with sleep and recovery with injury. Period. I didn't understand that regardless of your age or your level of athletic ability or training, everyone needs downtime. Until a few years ago, my days always began at high speed, and I essentially ran—or swam—through them, collapsing into bed at night. But in the last several years, as I've faced the reality of being an older athlete, I've learned that I just can't train as much as I did in my twenties without repercussions.

As I mentioned earlier, my joints hurt, I got injured more frequently, and I didn't have the stamina to train in the same way as all the teenagers and twenty-somethings in the pool. I realized, with the help of my coach at the time, that I needed to do less. At first, that was hard for me to understand and accept. Like any athlete worth her salt, I had always believed that working hard and training hard was the only way to be the best. But I would soon learn that not only was this not true, it was also self-defeating. I needed to learn how to rest.

It's taken me ten years to truly appreciate the wisdom of recovery as a regular and essential part of my training routine. As I mentioned in chapter 1, I first learned this lesson when I was training for the 2000 Olympics, working with my coach Richard Quick. He taught me the value of fewer laps and more intensity.

When I became pregnant with my daughter, Tessa, I learned even more about the power of rest and recovery. I was thirty-eight years old at the time. After so many years of trying to get pregnant, there was nothing that I wouldn't do to protect the baby. And when I started working out during my pregnancy (yes, it's true), I understood more fully what taking care of my body meant—because another one was growing inside of me.

The final phase of my learning this lesson came when I began training for the 2008 Beijing Olympics. By that point, I was thirty-nine years old. Many swimmers were now referring to me as "Mom," something I laughed at and got a kick out of. "I'll show them," I'd say silently to myself. And I did.

So it's taken me a number of years to *really* learn how to rest and recover, yet now it's probably the single most important dimension of my training regimen, a feature that has set me apart from many other elite-level athletes and helped me continue to train and perform at my peak.

Why Rest?

It makes sense that a body needs recovery time in order to perform at its best. Muscles need to rest in order to both avoid injury and build strength; bones, tendons, and ligaments need to realign with those muscles so they don't become overstretched or too tight; your skeleton needs to rebalance so that it maintains integrity; and even your brain needs a rest. When your body is given this opportunity, it will perform better for you. You will feel more balanced and more energetic, and experience a keener sense of overall well-being. It's a win-win.

Rest also helps you mentally and emotionally. We all know that feeling of being emotionally drained after receiving upsetting news, or of being exhausted and frazzled because of a stressful day or string of days. When I begin to feel weary, I know it's time to get extra sleep, carve out more downtime for myself, and try to have some fun. Rest means not working, not worrying—but it's up to you to figure out what helps you rest and relax most easily. Is it watching some of your favorite shows on TV? Is it reading a book curled up on your sofa? Is it playing in your garden, taking your dog for a walk, or going to the movies, where you can become completely absorbed without any interruptions from your daily life? One of the ways I love to kick back is going to get my nails done with Tessa. It's one of our favorite rituals: I get to spend girl time with my daughter in a completely relaxing, pampering way.

Pay Attention to Your Body

Recovery begins with paying attention to your body. This might sound simple, but when I was just beginning this process, I found it more difficult than I imagined because I was so used to feeling muscle pain, fatigue, and achiness in my joints. I'm not a complainer, so I figured I had to move through the pain, thinking that it would eventually go away. Right? Wrong.

If your body hurts, it's trying to tell you something. Pay attention to this message and see what you're doing that may be causing the cramping or the pulling or tugging feeling in a leg or shoulder and BACK OFF. For a long time I didn't pay attention to shoulder pain. I kept trying to work through it, and when I finally went to the doctor, it turned out I had a bone spur, which had caused a tear in my rotator cuff.

Be alert to signs of injury. As we age, our bodies are more tender and our ability to bounce back from injuries (minor or major) lessens. It becomes more important to key into an injury before it worsens. Here are some common signs of injury:

1. Pain in your joints, such as elbows, knees, ankles, or wrists.

2. Tenderness in a specific area, such as at the base of the neck, lower back, or feet.

3. Swelling. Inflammation is your body's natural defense against injury and indicates that your body is sending extra fluid to an area that is hurt or tired. Pay attention to this signal and back off.

When you are injured, you might want to use the classic **RICE** method for recovery.

R rest

I ice

C compression

E elevation

If you don't start to feel better in a couple of days, go see a doctor.

The Most Common Sports-Related Injuries

Following is a list of the most common sports- or workout-related injuries to watch for.

- **Achilles-tendon rupture:** The Achilles tendon is in the lower back of your calf and attaches your calf muscle to the bone. Tight or weak calf muscles can trigger Achilles tendonitis, which in turn can contribute to and/or cause a rupture.

- **Ankle sprain:** The most common of all ankle injuries, an ankle sprain occurs when there is a stretching and tearing of ligaments surrounding the ankle joint.

- **Anterior cruciate ligament (ACL) injury:** I know this one well. The ACL is located on the interior of your knee joint, attaching the femur bone to the tibia. This is the most common knee injury, with a partial or complete tear occurring when an athlete changes direction rapidly, twists without moving the feet, slows down abruptly, or misses a landing from a jump.

- **Blisters:** These little bubbles of skin are a nuisance but rarely deadly. You need to be careful when wearing new shoes, always wear socks, and if you do form blisters, make sure to keep the area clean so it doesn't get infected. You might recall that the reason I wear socks with my flippers during swim practice is to avoid blisters.

- **Concussion:** A concussion is typically caused by a severe head trauma, where the brain moves violently within the skull so that brain cells all fire at once, much like a seizure. If you think you might have hit your head and if there is any chance of a concussion, you need to go to the emergency room as quickly as possible.

- **Hamstring pull or tear:** Injuries to the hamstring are common among runners. The hamstring muscles run down the back of the leg from the pelvis to the lower leg bones, and an injury can range from minor strain to total rupture of the muscle.

- **IT band tightness:** The iliotibial band (the tendon that extends from the outer hip down the side of the quad) often gets tight and can cause pain if not stretched regularly.

- **Muscle cramps:** This sudden, tight, and intense pain is caused by a muscle locked in spasm.

- **Plantar fasciitis:** This is the most common cause of pain on the bottom of the heel, usually felt during the first steps of the morning.

- **Shin splints:** Experienced as pain in the front of the lower leg along the tibia (shin bone), shin splints are considered a cumulative stress injury.

- **Shoulder injury or fracture:** This typically is a total or partial break to either the clavicle (collarbone) or the neck of the humerus (arm bone). It generally is caused by an impact, such as a fall or blow to the shoulder.

- **Shoulder tendonitis, bursitis, or impingement:** These shoulder injuries (with which I am familiar) often occur together. If the rotator cuff and bursa (the inner lining of the shoulder, where muscle and bone meet) are irritated, inflamed, and swollen, they might become squeezed between the shoulder and the arm bone.

- **Stress fracture:** Stress fractures in the leg are often the result of overuse or repeated impacts on a hard surface.

- **Tendonitis:** A common sports injury, tendonitis, or inflammation of the tendons, often occurs from overuse and can cause deep, nagging pain.

- **Tennis elbow:** This injury is the number one reason people see their doctor for elbow pain. It is considered a cumulative trauma injury, meaning it occurs over time from repeated use of the muscles of the arm and forearm, which leads to small tears of the tendons.

- **Torn rotator cuff:** A common symptom of rotator-cuff injury is aching and weakness in the shoulder when the arm is lifted overhead.

If you think you might be suffering any one of these injuries, you should consult a physician or health-care provider for medical advice. Treatment options vary a great deal and can include surgery, medication (such as ibuprofen or a corticosteroid), chiropractic, RICE (see page 182), massage, and physical therapy.

Stay Hydrated

We're all told to drink at least eight glasses of water a day. But when you are training or working out, eight glasses is a bare minimum. It's absolutely mandatory that you replace your fluids after a workout, when you get up in the morning (everyone wakes up dehydrated and with low blood sugar), and before you go to bed.

How do you know if you're properly hydrated? One nutritionist told me to just watch the color of your urine: If it's dark yellow, then you need to drink more fluids. If it's almost clear with just a tinge of yellow, then your body is fine.

Dehydration not only causes cramping of the muscles and joints, it makes you feel light-headed and can lead to dizziness. It can creep up on you, so it's best to keep a water bottle on hand at all times.

When you rehydrate you are replacing not just fluids but electrolytes, including potassium, magnesium, sodium chloride, and calcium. When you work out, you upset the electrolyte balance that, for example, enables your muscles, to contract; if you don't restore the balance, you can experience muscle weakness.

I stay away from sports drinks—although they promise an electrolyte punch and other vitamins and minerals, they usually contain way too much sugar. I turn to them only if it's an emergency. Instead, I drink a lot of water. Sometimes VitaminWater, but I make sure it's the low-sugar variety. Remember, too, that some foods—especially fruits and vegetables—contain a lot of water. If you live near a Jamba Juice, grab one of their power fruit smoothies—and don't forget to add a shot of wheatgrass! (You'll know why when you get to chapter 8.)

Refuel Your Body

After a workout, it's important to refuel your body, especially with complex carbohydrates. Some experts speak about the "carb window," the sixty-minute period following a workout when your body needs

TORRES TIP

Post-workout Snack

My favorite post-workout snack is a perfect 1:4 ratio of protein to carbs: low-fat, organic chocolate milk. I also replenish with my Fitness Nutrition Amino Acids within twenty minutes after training. Pay attention to directions on the bottle.

carbs to replenish glycogen and your muscles can make this conversion three times faster than normal—in this way, you can refuel your body's energy resources, boost your metabolism, and burn fat.

One rule of thumb is to eat a snack with a 1:4 protein-to-carb ratio. One of my favorite snacks is low-fat, organic chocolate milk, which happens to have that 1:4 ratio. Other great snacks are a whole-grain bagel and cream cheese, peanut butter with apple or celery, banana smoothie with low-fat yogurt, or a handful of nuts and some dried cranberries.

Be wary of the energy bars that promise bountiful restoration but are high in calories, especially fat and sugars.

As I told you earlier, I have to eat frequently throughout the day—before my workout and after my workout as well as breakfast, lunch, and dinner. I don't like big meals (I just get too full and then uncomfortable) and prefer quick snacks that keep me feeling balanced. It might take some time and preparation, but try to figure out what you like to eat to refuel your body and how to have these snacks on hand so you don't skip this essential post-workout part of recovery.

Your Basic Recovery Plan

Here's an overview of how to approach post-workout recovery:

1. Replace your fluids.

2. Jump-start your glycogen replacement by eating a small meal or snack made up of mostly complex carbs.

3. Don't forget the protein to shore up amino acids used during exercise. The protein helps repair and refuel muscles.

Sleep, Baby, Sleep

Another rule of 8: All the science supports getting between seven and eight hours of sleep at night, with eight being recommended. Some people claim they just don't need that much sleep. But doctors and sleep experts will say that the body and brain need that much time to rest, to go through at least two REM cycles, to recharge the cells for metabolism, to boost immunity to fight off disease, and to decrease stress and fight the effects of aging.

When I'm just a few weeks out from a meet or other competition, I get more than eight hours of sleep—and if I don't, I'm a mess. I will take one-to-two-hour naps before big events just to keep my energy and balance. But most of the time, I'm in bed by ten and up at six-thirty or seven. When I travel across time zones, I make adjustments: If I go to the West Coast or Europe, I go to sleep a bit earlier and try to get up at my normal hour, so that in two or three days my body has adjusted to the time change. Before the 2008 Beijing Olympics, we actually arrived ten days in advance of the event so my body could acclimate to the change in time and recover from the long flight. Andy insists that for every hour of air travel, you need one day to recover.

When I'm under pressure from work, travel, or training, I try to take catnaps—even twenty minutes can be helpful. If Tessa goes down for a nap, I take this as a signal to rest, relax, or nap myself. Didn't we

TORRES TIP

Sleep Burns Fat

Did you know that recent research has shown that getting at least seven to eight hours of sleep each night boosts the metabolism and burns fat?

learn this from all those new-mom books? Nap when your child is napping? Postpartum, women's bodies need recovery—and they continue to need recovery time, just not as dramatically.

So when it comes to sleep, ask yourself these questions as a way to tune in to your current sleep habits:

1. Do you wake up feeling tired or well rested?

2. What time do you turn out the light?

3. Do you have trouble falling asleep? Does pre-bed television ever keep you awake because of high drama?

4. What is your sleep schedule like? Do you sleep less during the week and more on weekends? What's your pattern?

5. Is your bedroom dark, quiet, and cool? Do you think you'd sleep better with a sound machine?

We're all busy, trying to accomplish so much during the day, and we're accustomed to juggling many responsibilities. But your body and your brain need sleep. If you get into the habit of staying up too late, assuming you'll sleep in, you can trigger a bad sleep cycle. Try to go to bed at around the same time each night. And just as parents help their children go to sleep on their own by creating a bedtime ritual, create your own. Is it a cup of decaf tea? A warm shower or bath? Take your sleep seriously, so that you can get the most out of your night and your days. I've been known to have some warm milk before bed to settle me down.

TLC: Massage

If you can, get regular massages. I know this sounds extravagant—massages can get expensive—but there are ways around the cost and the benefits are enormous. For one, see if there are any massage schools in your area. Students learning this ancient healing art are always looking for subjects to work on—at a much lower fee than you'd pay normally.

For me, massages are a must. I get three forms of massage regularly. One is a technique called mashing that Steve and Anne do on me before races and on a regular basis for recovery. For me, mashing entails Steve and Anne using their feet and body weight (not all their body weight, but much more than they could summon using their hands) to pressure and knead the muscles of my legs, shoulders, abs, and arms. They vary the amount of pressure, but I like it pretty strong. I often use mashing as a pre-stretch routine to open and warm up my muscles.

I also enjoy Thai massage, which entails having a masseuse walk on my legs, belly, arms, shoulders, and back. It's more intense than a regular massage because of the use of the feet and more body weight. And I receive a special Swedish massage for my hands.

You can approximate mashing and/or Thai massage at home, with a partner or by yourself using foam rollers and other inexpensive equipment. The foam roller not only stretches muscles and tendons but also breaks down soft-tissue adhesions and scar tissue. By using your own body weight and a foam roller, you can perform a self-massage or myofascial release, break up trigger points, and soothe tight fascia while increasing blood flow and circulation to the soft tissues.

How Massage Works

The superficial fascia is a soft connective tissue located just below the skin. It wraps and connects the muscles, bones, nerves, and blood vessels. Together, muscle and fascia make up what is called the myofascia system. For various reasons including disuse, not enough stretching, or injuries, the fascia and the underlying muscle tissue can become stuck together. This is called an adhesion, and it results in restricted muscle movement. It also causes pain, soreness, and reduced flexibility or range of motion.

Myofascial release is a bodywork technique in which a practitioner uses gentle, sustained pressure on the soft tissue while applying traction to the fascia. This results in softening and lengthening (release) of the fascia and breaking down scar tissue or adhesions between skin, muscles, and bones. Myofascial release has also been shown to relieve various muscle and joint pains such as IT-band syndrome and shin splints, as well as improving flexibility and range of motion. Foam rollers are inexpensive, and with a bit of experimentation you can target just about any muscle group.

I know this sounds corny, but one of the ways that I know I'm relaxed and rested post-workout is if I can laugh and smile. If I find myself gripping the steering wheel or feeling short-tempered with anyone in my path, then I know I probably have not done enough of my recovery rituals. Again, recovery starts by paying attention to yourself—your body, your mood, your sleep patterns. Pay attention, and soon you'll know how to stop and take a deep breath; then you can reset your body.

8

PUTTING IT
TOGETHER

Congratulations! You have just completed reading about—if not doing—some of the most revolutionary strength and stretching techniques in fitness today! Now it's time to put it all together so that you can achieve the body you've always wanted—on the inside and out.

I hope that you've tried many of the individual strength and stretching movements and figured out at least one cardio workout that you enjoy, so that you have a sense of how much stronger, more energetic, and more confident you will feel practicing this approach to fitness. Now might be a good time to pause and think about how you really want to fit this workout into your life in a realistic way. You don't want these exercises to become part of a long list of been-there-done-that. You want to make sure that all that you've begun to learn about proper body alignment, biomechanics, and stretching and strengthening techniques will ground you, forming the foundation for how you approach fitness and health for the rest of your life.

Putting Together Your Workout

Think of your workout not as a single day but as a week overall. If you've decided that you can work out five days a week (a great goal to work toward, though often difficult to manage), then you can spread out the various components—cardio, strength, stretching, and recovery—throughout the week. If you're going to work out only three to four days a week, then you need to create a more intensely packed routine.

What is your main goal in trying this fitness plan? To lose weight? To sculpt your body? To increase lean muscle mass and lose fat? To increase your energy, sleep better, and look better? To train for a triathalon or optimize your performance for a particular sport? Only you can answer these questions and how you do will help you focus on your goals as you proceed.

Be realistic. What does your work schedule entail? What time do you go to bed, and how early do you wake up? Do you like to work out early in the day, before you face work or family responsibilities? Do you like to work out in the middle of the day, during a lunch break? Or do you prefer to work out in the evening, after work or after you've fed the kids? You need to decide on when you will work out in advance of the week. Also, I strongly recommend setting up a regular routine so that you don't have to rearrange your life on a day-to-day basis. Create your schedule and stick to it.

Figure out your cardio schedule. If you run, walk, or do something on your own, you have more freedom than if you're planning to do your cardio workout at a gym or in a fitness class. Make sure you know when the gym is open, when machines are least likely to be in use, and/or what the class schedule is.

Are you going to work out for a total of forty-five minutes, sixty minutes, or seventy-five minutes? How many days a week? Keep in mind that your week needs to include one-third strength training, one-third stretching (Ki-Hara), and one-third cardio, and of course time for recovery. As the workout routines below indicate, depending on how many days you work out, you will want to vary these components throughout the week.

The more often you work out the more quickly you will attain your goals, but you need to make sure that you cover all components and don't skimp on any one aspect. Try to work out a minimum of three days and a maximum of five days per week. As you will see below, the five-week workout plan is organized in three ways: based on three, four, or five days.

I swim (cardio) five days a week, for one and a half to two hours. I strength-train after my swim and stretch in the afternoon (sometimes twice a day if I'm approaching a meet or other competitive event). I actively recover seven days a week, and what I do varies—nap, get a massage, take a leisurely bike ride, go to the movies, or get my nails done with Tessa. The point of recovery is to relax and let your body repair itself. My days off are Thursday and Sunday. For those of you with a full-time job and a family, you might want to work out during the week, so you can relax on the weekends. Or do the opposite: work out once or twice during the week and once or twice more on the weekends, so you spread it throughout the week. Essentially, I tailor my workout for specific goals, paying close attention to how my body feels. If I begin to feel tight, I increase the stretching; if I feel exhausted, I back off and give myself more downtime; and if I feel weak, I increase the strengthening. As you put together your workout schedule, make sure you stay flexible in your head—and fit your workout to your needs.

The five-week plan will offer workouts on five days, but you can work out three days or four, if that's more suitable to your lifestyle. The bottom line is this: It's up to you to set your goals and push yourself in a way that makes sense—that is, create a healthy balance between pushing yourself and not overtraining.

Why five weeks? That's the classic time span for warming up your body, teaching it new movements, finessing technique, maximizing strength and endurance, and then finally realizing the results. Here's what it will look like:

Week One

The first week of any new exercise regimen is the hardest and the time when you're most prone to injury. During this initial period, you need to let your body warm up, pay special attention to how it feels, avoid overtraining, and know when to back off. Your focus is on your form so that you learn to execute any exercise in proper alignment.

Weeks Two and Three

The goal of these two weeks is to build strength and refine your technique, whether that's during a strength exercise, a resistance stretch, or a cardio workout. In this two-week block, you might increase the number of days you work out, lengthen your cardio time, or increase the reps of your strength and stretch exercises. Your body is now acclimated to the movements, so you will begin to feel stronger, and look leaner and more sinewy. This is also time to go inside of yourself. Get in touch with that inner athlete, reflect on your increasing confidence, self-assurance, and new level of energy. You might not need a boost from this well now, but in the next two-week period or on a day when you just can't get out of bed, you'll be more than grateful for this reserve of confidence.

Weeks Four and Five

Okay. I said the first week is the toughest, but this period comes in second. By week four, you will probably feel tired—that's good, you've-done-a-lot-to-deserve-it tired. However, if you stay focused on your technique, train just under your maximum, and make sure you recover religiously, this is the block of time that will generate the most visible, tangible re-sults in your body. Without a doubt you will be experiencing an increase in strength, you will feel more agile doing the exercises, and your perfor-mance will be enhanced during cardio or while playing a sport.

All of this is good. The hard part is that you might wake up and feel dead tired. You might find yourself writing a long list of to-dos, setting up an elaborate excuse for why you can't work out. You might think you've accomplished your goals, but this is when you go to that reserve of confidence. This is when you remind yourself of the com-mitment you made to *yourself.* This is when you get up and do it any-way. And I'll be there to help.

The Five-Week Blocks

Believe it or not, everyone, regardless of your previous strength-training experience, needs to start this workout plan with progression A of the strength training. Why? Because you need to do the strengthening movements for at least five weeks before you begin to see a return, in terms of both how you look and how you feel. It might take some of you even more than five weeks to see any visible results, such as more sinewy muscles, less adipose tissue, and more definition to your muscle groups. It also takes that long to learn the proper execution of the movements. So don't be in a hurry. Trust that these movements will ultimately de-liver the best results by setting you up to protect your alignment and teaching you how to do any strength-training exercise in proper form.

I've created a five-week workout plan based on the first progression of movements Andy designed. This is exactly where I started, even though I had been doing strength training with multiple coaches for more than twenty years before meeting Andy. So stick to the five-week plan for at least five weeks, before moving on to progression B and then C.

If at the end of the first five-week block you feel comfortable doing the movements, confident in your execution, and ready for more intensity, then you can substitute group B for A. You might also want to increase the intensity or duration of your cardio workout and double up on the Ki-Hara, doing all seventeen pairs of stretch strengtheners instead of splitting them into two groups within your week.

Essentially, you can stick with the original five-week plan for as long as you like. Move into the next two progressions once you feel you are ready but not before five weeks.

The five-week plan consists of four areas of fitness, so that a typical workout includes:

1. strength exercises

2. resistance stretching

3. cardio

4. recovery

Take a moment to create your exercise schedule:

DAY	TIME	ACTIVITY
Sunday		
Monday		
Tuesday		
Wednesday		
Thursday		
Friday		
Saturday		

Keep Your Workout Handy

I like to write up my workouts on a computer, print them out, and place them in a plastic sleeve that's easy to read and follow. I'm then able to take that with me to the gym, update the workout every five weeks or so, and then look back to former workouts quickly and easily.

As you become more familiar with the exercises and the flow of the workouts, you may fine-tune both your goals and your regimen. Perhaps you begin by working out three days each week but feel so good that you find one more day in your schedule to fit in another workout. Or maybe you start working out four days and find yourself just too tired by the end of the week—you then cut back to three days, which feels like enough for you.

Now let's get down to business!

The 5-Week Workout

PROGRESSION A

Five-Day Workout

	Day 1	Day 2	Day 3	Day 4	Day 5
Strength	For all movements, do 5 reps, 5 sets 1. Swiss Ball Cable Rotation (page 82) 2. Body-Weight Squat (page 88) 3. Dumbbell Incline Press (page 94) 4. Ground-Based Lat Pull-down (page 100) 5. Lateral Cable Walk-out (page 106)		For all movements, do 5 reps, 5 sets 1. Swiss Ball Cable Rotation (page 82) 2. Body-Weight Squat (page 88) 3. Dumbbell Incline Press (page 94) 4. Ground-Based Lat Pull-down (page 100) 5. Lateral Cable Walk-out (page 106)		For all movements, do 5 reps, 5 sets 1. Swiss Ball Cable Rotation (page 82) 2. Body-Weight Squat (page 88) 3. Dumbbell Incline Press (page 94) 4. Ground-Based Lat Pull-down (page 100) 5. Lateral Cable Walk-out (page 106)
Stretch		Ki-Hara 1 to 8 + bonus (page 154)		Ki-Hara 9 to 16 + bonus (page 154)	
Cardio		30 to 45 minutes		30 to 45 minutes	
Recovery	15 to 20 minutes	15 to 20 minutes	1 hour	15 to 20 minutes	15 to 20 minutes

Four-Day Workout

	Day 1	Day 2	Day 3	Day 4
Strength	For all movements, do 5 reps, 5 sets 1. Swiss Ball Cable Rotation (page 82) 2. Body-Weight Squat (page 88) 3. Dumbbell Incline Press (page 94) 4. Ground-Based Lat Pull-down (page 100) 5. Lateral Cable Walk-out (page 106)		For all movements, do 5 reps, 5 sets 1. Swiss Ball Cable Rotation (page 82) 2. Body-Weight Squat (page 88) 3. Dumbbell Incline Press (page 94) 4. Ground-Based Lat Pull-down (page 100) 5. Lateral Cable Walk-out (page 106)	
Stretch		Ki-Hara 1 to 8 + bonus (page 154)		Ki-Hara 9 to 16 + bonus (page 154)
Cardio	45 minutes		45 minutes	
Recovery	15 to 20 minutes	15 to 20 minutes	15 to 20 minutes	15 to 20 minutes

Three-Day Workout

	Day 1	Day 2	Day 3
Strength	For all movements, do 5 reps, 5 sets 1. Swiss Ball Cable Rotation (page 82) 2. Body-Weight Squat (page 88) 3. Dumbbell Incline Press (page 94) 4. Ground-Based Lat Pull-down (page 100) 5. Lateral Cable Walk-out (page 106)		For all movements, do 5 reps, 5 sets 1. Swiss Ball Cable Rotation (page 82) 2. Body-Weight Squat (page 88) 3. Dumbbell Incline Press (page 94) 4. Ground-Based Lat Pull-down (page 100) 5. Lateral Cable Walk-out (page 106)
Stretch	Ki-Hara 1 to 16 + bonus (page 154)	Ki-Hara 1 to 16 + bonus (page 154)	Ki-Hara 1 to 16 + bonus (page 154)
Cardio	30 to 45 minutes	30 to 45 minutes	30 to 45 minutes
Recovery	15 to 20 minutes	15 to 20 minutes	15 to 20 minutes

PROGRESSION B

After you've completed at least one five-week block of Progression A, you might feel ready to tackle the next progression in Andy's strength-training approach. As you may recall from chapter 4, progression B increases in complexity, range of motion, degree of difficulty (in terms of execution), and intensity.

Depending on the frequency of your workout (three, four, or five days), simply replace the strength exercises in progression A with those in progression B:

PROGRESSION B STRENGTHENERS

1. Fixed Medicine Ball Rotation Pass (page 84)

2. BOSU Dumbbell Squat (page 90)

3. Smith Press Crunch (page 96)

4. Single-Arm Cable Row Twist (page 102)

5. Side-Bridge Cable Row (page 108)

TORRES TIP

Relax Your Resting Muscles

Muscles are either on or off. There is no in between—either your muscles are firing and contracted, using energy, or they are not. There's no such thing as kind of contracted. Get to know your muscles, and pay attention to what muscles you need when. If you're familiar with the muscles your body is using, you can relax the muscles you're not using. Learn to relax!

PROGRESSION C STRENGTHENERS

Once you have achieved a level of intensity, performance, and execution with progression B, you might be ready for an even more intense challenge. Here is progression C of Andy's strength-training approach:

1. Alternating Cable Squat Rotation (page 86)

2. Rainbow with Medicine Ball (page 92)

3. Bench Plyo Push-up (page 98)

4. Cable Push-Pull Rotation (page 104)

5. Star Push-up (page 110)

||||||||||||||||||||||||||||||||||||||||||||||||||||||||||||||||||||||||||||||||||||||||

Torres Tips for Recovery

Remember, recovery means time away from working out to let your body refuel, rest, and recuperate; it's physical, mental, emotional, and social. Here's a quick list of ways to recover:

Physical

Rehydrate your body with fluids

Replenish amino acids

Replace electrolytes

Get a massage

Take a hot soak or whirlpool bath

Walk in the woods

Cardio Ideas

As I stressed in chapter 6, including cardio in your regular routine is a must, but how you choose to do a cardio workout is entirely up to you. I clock most of my cardio swimming, but I do like to add some variety and make it fun. I love to roller-skate, bike, and if I'm at the beach, I'll take a run (because of creaky knees, I can only tolerate running on surfaces that provide a lot of give).

Cardio should be fun! Of course, when it's an activity you enjoy, you are more likely to do it. If you simply like to walk, then simply walk! But you've got to try a few things in order to find one, two, or three that you like.

Varying your cardio is important. If you go to a gym and you're used to using the elliptical machine for your cardio workout, great. But there might come a day when you find yourself wanting to skip your cardio because you're bored. That's when you have to have an arsenal of other activities that you can turn to so you can keep moving!

Here is a quick reference list so you don't forget all your options:

Elliptical or treadmill

Swimming

Step class

Running

Tennis/squash

Dance class (Zumba or Nia)

Roller-skating/ice-skating/Rollerblading

Biking/cycling/spin class

Cross-country skiing (in winter obviously!) or NordicTrack

Nap

Make sure you're getting at least seven to eight hours of sleep

Mental

Yoga

Read a good book

Zone out to a favorite television show

Listen to music

Go to the movies

Emotional and Social

Get together with friends for coffee or a meal

Go dancing!

Reconnect with an old friend via e-mail or Facebook

Spend time with your family

Although you need to physically recover after any workout by replenishing and rehydrating your body (see page 185 for more details), the amount of recovery time does vary throughout the week. I know it's never easy to find this "me" time, so I've suggested trying to fit in fifteen to twenty minutes—touching base with yourself for even this amount of time can give you a chance to relax and destress. And on two days each week (midweek and at the start of a new week), you will benefit from at least one hour of time that is completely stress-free. Whether you spend that time alone relaxing or with family and friends is up to you. What's important is that you allow yourself time to unwind and let your body reset itself. You will not only feel stronger

Don't Forget to Warm Up!

Before any workout, remember to do a quick, five-minute warm-up—even if it's a five-minute light jog on the treadmill. You need to warm up your body and get the blood moving to all your muscles. Take it slow, and pay attention to how your body feels. If something feels tight, keep that in mind as you begin your workout, and make an adjustment if necessary. For instance, if you notice that your quads are tight, you might want to do extra stretches to help loosen them during your resistance stretching.

when you do return to your regular workout, you will maximize the results from the workouts already done!

What Are the Benefits of Your Workout?

Increase your cardiovascular health and fat-burning ability

Increase your body's ability to build and maintain muscle mass

Increase and hold on to bone density

Strengthen your body's immune system and ability to fight illness

Train for sport performance

Have the ability to enhance/change your mood/emotional out-look in an instant

At this point you might need to touch base with your goals again. Do you need to ramp them up? Ease them? Do you feel good and want to continue just as you're doing? You are the one who knows best. Trust yourself. The more familiar you are with the individual movements, and the more regular your routine becomes, the more trust you will have in your own judgment and assessment of yourself. But just know that when you follow good form and execution, when you take the time to recover on all fronts—body, mind, and heart—then you'll take your body's health and physical prowess to new levels, sharpen your mental focus, and reach new performance heights.

Getting fit is all about reaching for, achieving, and sustaining a commitment to taking care of yourself for the rest of your life. You might need to make adaptations—to keep feeding surprises to your body and mind just to keep things fun. But change does not mean stopping or giving up. By the time you complete one five-week block, I promise that not only will you miss exercise when you miss a workout, but both your body and mind will need to work out to feel good. You're at a place where fitness feels like "I get to!" instead of "I have to!"

SOME FINAL THOUGHTS

||||||||||||||||||||||||||||||||||||||||||||||||||||||||||||||||||||||||||||||||||||||||||||||||||||||||||||||||||||||||||||

I'm a mother, a daughter, a sister, an aunt, and a friend, but being an athlete is a huge part of my identity. And it will always be. I think this vision of myself, even if I had not made two comebacks after the age of thirty, has kept me young in spirit, vital in mind and body, and always open to change. Being an athlete is in essence how I best take care of myself, how I stay connected to my desire to win, how I seek out and find challenges in my life that enable me to keep growing as a person.

I can't imagine my life without a high physical component driving me through my days because I know it's the way that I create the energy and confidence to tackle any job, accomplish any goal. And I think fitness can do the same for you. In this way, getting into shape and staying fit is both a lifestyle choice and a commitment to taking care of yourself, inside and out.

The first step is to take your fitness seriously. Have fun, for sure. But make a commitment to yourself: Try this workout plan for five weeks. And when you finish that five weeks, give it another five weeks.

Maybe you have to go to bed earlier; maybe you have to learn to be more efficient at work; maybe you have to say no to a child's request to take her to the mall. There are things in your life you can give up when you make fitness a priority.

What I think you will find is that the more active you are, the better you will be at what you do. You will think more clearly and quickly, you will move through your day without hesitation. As your body gets stronger and in better shape, you are naturally going to feel more confident. You will walk more upright, you will move with more self-assurance, and you will act with more deliberation. Day-to-day tasks will feel effortless, and work will feel good, not like something you dread. You will begin to think of yourself as strong in all ways. You're also going to look better and feel better, and we all know that boosts confidence.

When these changes begin to happen, they are signs that you are connecting to your inner power source. This is true body-mind connection. And when you start connecting with that inner place, the world is your oyster.

I hope these workouts will inspire you to make fitness a priority in your life. You are in charge. If you try these workouts and stick with them, you will see your body become lean and strong, you will feel your energy mount and your focus sharpen, and you will be able to accomplish whatever it is that you desire. You've got what it takes to make your dreams real, you just have to believe. That's the heart of *Gold Medal Fitness*—now go for the gold!